BODY, MIND, & EMOTIONAL WORK FOR ANXIETY

Complementary Healing Approach for Concentration Loss, Tension All Over & Not Getting Enough Sleep

Holistic Healing for Beginners Series

P. RESTAINO

We hope you benefit from the complementary medicine presented.
Remember tracking what helps you feel healthy is important.

If you feel inspired to leave a review we would appreciate your kind words.
http://amazon.com/review/create-review?asin=+B09TYM79TN

Drop us an email or stop by our website:

support@choosinggoodness.com

www.choosinggoodness.com

Another book by Choosing Goodness:

What Makes Me Feel Better? How I Am Getting Healthy Workbook

This book is dedicated to all the holistic healers around the world,

thank you for sharing your gift.

I am exceedingly grateful to all who have touched me,

so I can heal myself in preparation to heal others.

CONTENTS

INTRODUCTION

If you are one of hundreds of millions of people that suffer from anxiety and stress, know that you are not alone. The person who understands your challenges best is YOU! This is a go-to book for you to learn more about alternative medicine as a tool to manage your anxiety in a holistic way. We compiled twelve complementary healing approaches so you can choose what makes you feel empowered and feel most vibrant.

This book was created to offer you options to break through your issues, to respond to your anxiety, with tools that are appropriate for various situations. We trust your judgement. and are not encouraging you to disregard medical professionals, we are presenting complementary approaches for you to manage your anxiety. After reading this book, you will be knowledgeable of techniques and information to go forth and create a new path for your life. Overcome frustration from the vicious clutches of anxiety. You can choose which tools give you the power to make necessary changes to break the bonds of anxiety and live relaxed.

Our intention in designing this book is to give you an overview of each alternative approach to expand your understanding, the benefits of each modality, and examples of how a person utilized this complementary approach to become a happier and healthier individual. Those who finish reading this book will gain a sense of empowerment, to choose what changes they decide to integrate, to improve their life.

Throughout this book we will use the terminology that we would like to clarify. The term 'modality' is a word we use for each technique presented in this book, it is defined as "a type of treatment for a disease or medical condition" (Cambridge, 2021). "Alternative, Complementary, Integrative, and Holistic, we use interchangeably. Alternative refers to modalities that did not originate within the contemporary medical structure. Complementary and integrative indicate the manner in which an alternative modality easily complements or integrates with contemporary western medicine. Holistic is a term that insinuates the whole being is taken into consideration - body, mind, spirit, and emotions. This is the basis for most alternative medicine." (Frisch, 2001) Healing refers to the process of becoming healthy. All of the approaches in this book are referred to as medicine. We strongly believe you can be hopeful integrating holistic healing rather than pharmaceutical solutions. Take time to learn more about yourself so you are comfortable taking charge of your wellbeing.

The medical profession has clinical definitions for anxiety, we believe describing a technical perspective does not honor you, the person struggling to live a joyful life. You know what anxiety feels like or you would not be reading this book. The unfortunate truth is that constant anxiety often transcends the mental and emotional side of things and can seep into physical ailments too. This may cause a lack of sleep, concentration loss, illness, racing mind, or even mental diseases and disorders. It often causes muscle tension, hinders the functioning of the immune system, and keeps those suffering from enjoying their life. The constant feeling of being overwhelmed can result in panic, some of us are too scared to even leave our own homes. These realities are our concern and a motivation for providing holistic healing tools for you to consider, as you pursue a healthier life.

Anxiety may always be with you in one way or another, complementary medicine holds a multitude of benefits. On a psychological, mental, and emotional level, alternative healing has positive effects such as enhancing the ability to focus, concentrate, improve memory, balance your emotions, uplift self-awareness, and confidence. On a physical level, holistic healing can provide relief by assisting with pain management. It also decreases levels of fatigue you may feel from high anxiety. It can further reduce the sensations of muscle tension and stiff joints, often increasing mobility and heightening energy levels. Alternative healing can help improve sleeping patterns and assist in mitigating insomnia. It further strengthens the immune system. Certain techniques are known to shed unnecessary burdens from your nervous system, resulting in improved digestion, which is closely related to the body's production of serotonin. More of this pleasure-producing hormone combats the anxiety producing the hormone cortisol.

The origin of anxiety is an evolutionary trait present in all humans, passed on from our hunter-gatherer ancestors. Millions of years ago, homo sapiens lived in the wild where there were many life-or-death threats to face constantly. An instinctive fight-or-flight response ultimately saved humanity and helped us evolve into the species we are today. Our minds still latch onto modern-day problems that initiate this innate fight-or-flight response.

These days we are ruled by technology, which has caused a global disconnect from nature and organic life. Social media has heightened unrealistic standards and those of us who check our social media pages are constantly faced with a mixture of reactions. We can feel as though we are not good enough, we often judge or compare as we see all the emojis being posted at any moment of the day or night. Add the stress of Covid-19, the unknown factor of who may be infected next and how it is changing our lives and causing deaths around the world. Plus, the amount of information we process now includes: catastrophic situations occurring across the world, such as genocide, wars, earthquakes, hurricanes, all while we're often stuck in a stressful job to pay the rent. We are constantly managing an explosion of sensory overstimulation: bright lights, loud noises, uncertain chemicals in our food, water, or air. Changes are happening at the speed of light and the evolution of our brain understandably struggles to catch up.

Our physical reaction is the release of a hormone called cortisol. Too much of this hormone can have detrimental and long-lasting effects, causing actual disorders or mental limitations that hinder our ability to function with ease. Because our triggers differ by individual it makes sense that treatment may be different for each person, at different times of life. This is another reason we are offering so many alternative methods in one book.

All in all, anxiety is plaguing the world right now. According to the Anxiety & Depression Association of America "Today, anxiety disorders are the most common mental illness in the U.S., affecting 40 million adults in the United States (Facts & Statistics, n.d.). Around the world 300 million people have a type of anxiety disorder, as reported by The World Health Organization.

Alongside the rise of our anxiety prone lifestyles, pharmaceutical corporations took over providing an instant solution. The first appearance of Western medicine was seen as miraculous. More lives were saved and many deaths prevented with vaccines. The population was growing, and we were gaining access to many quick fixes that calmed the symptoms. Often, society starts with great intentions related to drugs, or other inventions, yet the best laid plans have a tendency to go astray. For example, opioids were intended to assist in treating pain and became a commonly used treatment in the Civil War era. There have been different types of opioids for pain that were created with an intent to be less addictive over the years, yet we are still facing an opioid addiction epidemic (The Origin and Causes of the Opioid Epidemic, 2018). According to the U.S. Department of Health and Human Service in 2019 there were 70,630 opioid overdose deaths, 10.1 million people misusing their prescriptions, 1.6 million people were diagnosed with an opioid use disorder (What is the U.S. Opioid Epidemic?, 2021). However, we invite you to consider that long lasting holistic approaches can solve our issues starting from the root cause.

Holistic healing encompasses alternative medicine that does not involve pharmaceuticals. These integrative methods focus on a body as a whole, taking into account the mind, emotions, and spirit. The basis of these modalities emphasize identifying the root cause instead of numbing the symptoms and side effects. The holistic philosophy is aimed at restoring balance, promoting harmony, and energy flow across all levels of a human being. Alternative medicine varies in type, some were developed thousands of years ago withstanding the harsh tests of time. Others were founded in the 20th century offering new approaches to older philosophies. The prevalence and popularity of these holistic methods only further prove their effectiveness.

Being trained in Healing Touch, I completed level 5 and am a Practitioner Apprentice. As part of the certification, I experienced more than 10 different modalities, to gain a better understanding of other holistic therapies being offered. At that time, I realized how diverse and valuable complementary medicine is. As my healing capacity expanded so did my appreciation for all those who honorably choose to heal people and this planet in different ways. Additionally, I attended three 13 Indigenous Grandmothers gatherings which broadened my exposure to traditional medicine that has enhanced lives for centuries. My experience with traditional medicine increased as I went to Peru and spent time with the Achual tribe and assisted friends, born in Mexico and living in California, with ceremonies. I feel blessed to be able to contribute to people regarding their health and wellness. These experiences made it clear, it is not my place to tell anyone how they are to become healthier, it is to offer information and encourage them to use natural alternatives first. I trust everyone will make the best decision for themselves, so we all enjoy healthier lives. The greatest gift I received from "...healing is about letting go of expectations and ego, and connecting to others with our Divine Essence" (Healing Beyond Borders (HBB) Education Committee, 2010).

There are numerous types of complementary medicine, we discuss twelve within this book. We are not implying a modality that is not covered in this compilation, is inferior in any way. The intention of this book is to expose you to a variety of alternative options, to help you consider the value, and realize they offer legitimate options, while opening your mind to holistic medicine. If you are drawn to an integrative approach, such as Acupuncture, we encourage you to pursue healthy options that work to help you reduce your anxiety.

Here is a brief summary of what is included in this book: First, we take a look at Laughter Therapy, which is aimed at increasing levels of serotonin and an overall sense of calm and happiness in life. The second chapter focuses on Aromatherapy and the use of powerful essential oils to soothe the mind and bring forth a heightened sense of mental awareness. The third chapter tackles the history, science, and effectiveness of Emotional Freedom Tapping (EFT) demonstrating how certain tapping points on the body can induce feelings of calm and relax the body as a whole. Following this is an in-depth look at exercise and how movement can be an impactful form of medicine to heal the ever racing mind. Then we move onto the ancient, sacred, elaborate practice of Ayurveda which offers meditation, yoga, bathing, Panchakarma treatments that incorporate herbs. Animal Therapy in chapter six helps us gain a deeper understanding of the healing gift of animals and the bonds humans can form with pets as companions. Chapter seven introduces energy work in the form of Healing Touch and Reiki, how it works, and how it can help ease sensations of stress and anxiety by aligning our chakras so energy flow takes charge and we heal ourselves. Continuing on we move into Sound Healing and the scientific explanations of vibrations and frequencies, which can significantly impact and alter our physical and emotional states for the better. Finally, the last chapter takes us on a journey through Hypnotherapy, an extremely effective tool to help one heal from deeper trauma and create new, healthier, and long-lasting habits.

Being able to evaluate how advantageous any treatment is for you, is a critical aspect of your health. In addition to each chapter providing reflection questions at the end, consider using the addendum to create your personalized tracking system. You will find in-depth examples and guidance so you can decide what is most important to measure, as you learn what reduces your anxiety. Consider using the companion workbook *What Makes Me Feel Better?* Then you can track if there are benefits for any given medicine you choose. Learning more about yourself, tracking your triggers, your reactions, as well as what calms you, can be the most valuable tool of a healthier life.

Use this book as a resource to truly realize your potential and see it through. With every page you turn, you can evaluate different techniques to be an uplifted, happier, and healthier version of you. Take the leap of faith into this daunting process, make the decision to help yourself. If you have tried many options, never give up. Be proud of empowering yourself with new possibilities for life. We commend your efforts and are excited to welcome you with open arms to embrace the world of Complementary Healing. Let's take a journey to learn which tools you want to break the bonds of anxiety, so you can enjoy the good life.

CHAPTER ONE

— : —

LAUGHING WITH ANXIETY

Let's start with the easiest modality to incorporate into your life that helps manage anxiety, Laughter! Holistically your body, mind, heart and spirit are affected from laughing. The sense that is most impacted by this approach is hearing. In this chapter you will learn about how easy it is to share with friends, the medical benefits of laughter, gain access to tips on ways to incorporate laughter into your life, and be challenged to decide how you might incorporate this technique into your daily actions.

Introducing Laughter as Medicine

The saying that laughter is the best medicine, has been proven to be true through research studies and stories. There is a foundation in Ireland called the Havin' a Laugh Charity that works to find ways to overcome mental health struggles through life enhancing activities and laughter. They even put out a book of funny stories, jokes, poems, art, and more, to ignite laughter and uplift people. This charity was born after several founding members lost loved ones to mental illness (About Us, 2021).

According to Science Direct there has been an increase to anxiety and depression recently due to the Covid-19. Recent studies have shown this pandemic has made a substantial impact causing a three fold increase of depression in the U.S.A. While this is an ongoing issue laughter was listed as an intervention therapy to help alleviate these anxiety and depression symptoms. In a meta-analysis on 814 participants from 10 published studies, laughter interventions were reported to significantly reduce depression and anxiety levels, along with an increase in better quality of sleep; the benefits on depression were more pronounced with long-term laughter intervention (Akimbekov & Razzaque, 2021).

Benefits of Laughter Therapy

Laughter therapy, a form of rehabilitation that utilizes the act of laughing to decrease stress, is now often harnessed to help treat anxiety and depression. But it's not just your face that is doing the work. Laughter exercises involve the entire body, both within and on the outside. It touches on mental, physical, spiritual, and emotional aspects of the body and mind as they have a constant connection. What happens to the physical body can have a deep effect on the mental part of the body, too. When you start laughing, even if you're forcing yourself do it initially, your mind automatically assumes something of excitement or joy is occurring and instantly releases chemicals that support your mood for the better. By creating good feelings within the physical body, you're reflecting the positive energies into the brain.

Laughter therapy involves a mix of physical exercises that can trigger the body's laughter reaction. The tossing of the arms, the long strides of the legs, and the diaphragm exercises all contribute to a positive sense of emotions. Even the very simple act of making yourself laugh, especially when you don't feel like it, can have profound effects on the mind. The brain doesn't actually know whether you are laughing for real or faking it; therefore, the brain releases chemicals and has the same effect on the body as real laughing does. This helps in making the conscious choice to try to uplift your current mood and also aids in an overall increased mood.

Humor, laughing, and smiling can bring us joy, happiness, and a sense of peace. Laughter aids in a deeper connection to those around you, lightens the heavy burden you may be carrying on your shoulders, and unearths a sense of hope. It also acts as an energy releaser. Humans experience various different things in a single day, many of which can alter their perception and change their level of anxiety. However, dwelling on negative experiences and emotions can cause energy to be stored within the body. This energy needs to be released in order to fully release anxious emotions. Laughter is a way to release this energy, thus making you feel lighter, less restricted, and less stressed.

Laughter is incredibly good for you in various ways. It physically relaxes the body, helping relieve tension; it boosts the immune system through the decrease of stress hormones and increases antibodies which battle infections and diseases; and it boosts the production and transportation of endorphins within the bloodstream, instantly increasing your mood. Laughter also keeps your heart safe and healthy as it boosts the strength and functioning of blood vessels and flow. But while it has tremendous effects on the physical aspects of the body, it also has seemingly endless benefits on the mind. It halts anxious, sad, or distressing emotions; increases energy and mental clarity; shifts perspectives toward a healthier, logical, and more positive approach; and, as mentioned before, cultivates bonds between people.

Laughter yoga, laughter therapy, and act of laughing itself, is becoming a widespread phenomenon. It's completely free, requires absolutely no tools, and can be done any time at any place. From the Philippines and India to America and South Africa, laughter yoga and therapy is making waves with millions of smiles across the globe. While anxiety, stress, and depression are no joke, laughter can help mitigate the effects and emotions derived from irritability and anxiety.

The Science of Laughter

As human beings, we all face a level of anxiety. It is seemingly hard wired in our genetics from millions of years of having to survive the harsh reality we find ourselves. Sometimes, anxiety can help us navigate danger and save us. However, too much anxiety can be crushing and almost paralyzing. When we reach this level of stress, it can be extremely difficult to get ourselves out of this dark space. However, there are holistic ways of dealing with this, such as laughter therapy. We have already explored the benefits of laughing, so now, we can discover how it actually works on a more scientific basis.

The region of the brain that causes anxiety and stress is the amygdala, which is responsible for processing negative emotions. Alternatively, the region of the brain that deciphers pleasure is the frontal cortex, an area that also functions as the decision maker. This directly relates to the fact that when we ease our anxiety with laughter, we're able to immediately shift our perspective and let go of the more emotional effects. This act of mindset adjustment is called the reappraisal effect. It works through a specific concept. It is not the situation that is negative or harmful but rather the thought aspect of the situation. Your mind is extremely powerful and you actually have more control over it than you may think. Through simple exercises like laughing, we can assist ourselves with helping our brain conduct a more positive perspective. Even Freud, one of the world's most famous psychologists, believed that laughing can heal through the release of stored energy and provide a break from the seemingly ever-worrying mind.

For thousands of years, the act of laughter has been directly linked to one's well-being and can have a direct influence on our health. Thus, laughter is used to:

- Bolster health, both physically and mentally

- Relieve tension in your brain

- Decrease stress hormones

- Release healthy chemicals called endorphins, which act to mitigate the brain's very perception of pain itself

- Cause enlightenment, following the chemical theory

Additionally, laughter influences and controls specific parts of the brain plus the entire bodily system as a whole. It involves the respiratory, immune, muscular, nervous, endocrine, and cardiovascular system. Laughing exercises are known to:

- Relax the muscles, easing tension.

- Bolster respiration and trigger blood circulation, bringing more oxygen to the brain and helping curate a clearer mind, improving both memory and mental clarity

- Decrease stress hormones, thus increasing your overall mood, self-esteem, and energy

- Elevate and uplift the immune system, contributing to an overall healthy physical state

The therapy of laughter focuses on the mental aspect and how working toward an enlightened psychological effect can positively influence the entire body. Laughing lessens the levels of epinephrine and cortisol—the serums responsible for anger and fear—and metabolic regulation and inflammation respectively. Laughter, therefore, reverses the very effects of these serums, thus reversing the chemical influence of stress.

Depression is often associated with anxiety. It attacks the brain in a completely different way. However, laughter can also be used as a tool to help fight this mental battle, but we first need to share an introduction to what depression is, to fully conceptualize why laughter can help mitigate the desperate influence of depression. Depression is not just a state of mind but an actual clinical disease. It occurs when the neurotransmitters within the brain are reduced. These include serotonin, dopamine, and norepinephrine, transmitters that are responsible for pleasure and happiness. Without the full functioning of these vital neurotransmitters, the entire mind and body will be weakened, causing an individual to experience depression. Laughter is used to promote a healthy release of serotonin and dopamine in the bloodstream, brain, and body. As mentioned before, even if you fake or force laughter, your brain cannot tell the difference and releases these essential positive neurotransmitters. Therefore, through the act of laughing, whether it is genuine or not, you can send an increased amount of pleasure hormones to the brain and fight the depressive disease.

In a more general approach, laughter aids in bonding people together and strengthening relationships, helping you feel supported and loved. Humans both need and long for connection, and often, those struggling with depression feels isolated and alone. By curating a routine of laughter and experiencing it with others, you can satisfy this desire for connection, feeling a sense of achievement, purpose, and belonging. This not only fights the sensation of loneliness, hopelessness, and anxiety, it helps you navigate depression and boosts self-confidence while increasing your ability to relate with others.

To sum it up, laughter really can be the best form of medicine in some cases. On a physical level, laughter increases your oxygen intake, which, in turn, supports the functioning of your heart, lungs, and muscles. Furthermore, laughter relaxes one's muscles, relieving physical tension and helping you lighten up. Laughter also boosts the immune system through the release of antibodies that fight diseases and infections. It releases endorphins that halt the production and transportation of stress hormones which then lowers blood pressure. Add to that, the fact laughter burns calories, further uplifting your self-confidence and self-esteem. It improves your mood through the reduction of stress hormones and the increase of serotonin and dopamine, and it also strengthens your relationship with others which combats feelings of loneliness.

Getting Better Every Day

Laughter can have profound positive effects on those suffering from anxiety or depression. However, in order to fully experience the numerous physical and mental benefits of laughter, it needs to be woven into your daily or weekly routine. While this may sound daunting to add another task to your list, laughter is extremely easy and will help you uplift your entire life for the better. Consider these suggestions:

1. Start by simply smiling more - It triggers the pleasure response in your brain, and it is very contagious, allowing you to spread your joy to others and cast a brighter light on the world. Smile at people who pass you in the street, smile when you're basking in the glorious sunshine, or smile at yourself in the mirror when you're brushing your teeth. Notice the influence you can have on others as well as yourself.

2. Practice Gratitude - Another extremely simple yet effective way to smile and laugh. Every morning share with yourself or others a few things you are grateful for. This can be having a roof over your head, being supportive, food on the table, legs that let you walk, a voice that lets you speak, or something beautiful surrounding you. By making a conscious effort to count your blessings—and continuing to do so— you can rewire your brain to start seeing what's positive wherever you are, no matter what situation you are in. This will also help you smile and laugh, diminishing your anxiety around your problems and helping you realize that life may be a bit better than you may have previously thought.

3. If you see or hear laughter, get involved - People are usually more than happy to share their happiness, jokes, and laughter with others. Engage in these conversations and even dare to contribute. This not only helps you laugh and smile more yourself but will aid in bringing you closer to others and forming more solid connections. In the same breath, start spending more time with those who make you laugh, anyone who truly understands your humor.

4. Encourage simulated laughter (laughter that is not spontaneous but rather forced). - Laughter yoga and laughter therapy are

ways to do it and one of the most effective ways at that. Laughter Yoga is used to incorporate laughter exercises with yoga breathing techniques. You can find this in social laughter clubs, companies and corporations that provide classes, yoga studios, colleges, universities (Laughter Yoga Health Craze Sweeping the World, 2021). One simple approach is to set a timer for 60 seconds and start laughing. The more you do it the easier it gets. Often, once an individual begins in a group, it becomes contagious, and everyone laughs with each other. We promise in 60 seconds your mind will have a new perspective. Many classes will begin with breathing techniques, clapping or chanting such as "ho-ho, ha-ha" leading to you letting loose, laughing and enjoying yourself (Davidson, 2021).

5. If you're looking for ways to invite more genuine and spontaneous laughter into life - There are many things you can start undertaking today. This includes watching funny movies, comedy shows, or YouTube videos, reading funny books or comic strips, spending more time with people you find humorous, hosting fun and exciting game nights, engaging in activities you may find amusing such as karaoke, and finding the comedy in things and people around you.

6. Place reminders of things that bring you humor, joy, and smiles in your space - This can be a poster or picture that makes you laugh, a photo of a heartfelt and fun memory, listening to a comedy podcast during your work break, or writing funny or inspiring comments on a mirror with erasable colored pens.

Invite laughter into every aspect of your life. Be curious and seek out the humor in situations. Attend laughter therapy and laughter yoga to bolster the benefits and to experience an overall improvement in both your physical and mental well-being.

Reflection

Now that you have more information describing laughter and its benefits to reduce anxiety, take a moment to decide if you want to take action or place laughter on hold. Laughter can be an alternative medicine that benefits many, we hope you are one.

- Is Laughter Therapy a tool you want to use in your life?

- Are you ready to include laughter as part of a reduce anxiety Self Care program now?

- Write down which of the recommendations you can integrate into your life.

- Specify which days of the week and time of day there is a bit of time in your schedule, to increase your laughter. Would you prefer to laugh alone or with others?

- What will you measure to see if this modality is helping to manage your anxiety?

Notes & things to remember....

CHAPTER TWO

— · —

AROMATHERAPY SCENTS HELP ANXIETY

*The next modality is about Essential oils and aromatherapy
because they shift our nervous system through the sense of
smell. This can be a gentle method to manage anxiety. Start
simple as some people have allergies to scents. Those who
have the freedom to smell often enjoy this unassuming yet
impactful holistic approach. This chapter will share a story of
how a businesswoman was able to shift foggy brain to include
aromatherapy throughout her life. Also included are benefits
of essential oil, a list of plant oils and their potential impact,
and encouragement to decide if you might incorporate this
technique into your anxiety healing tools.*

A Story About Aromatherapy

One day, Los Angeles entertainment executive Carla Cohen woke up
feeling starkly strange. Her brain was foggy, she felt endlessly fatigued,

and she had no clue what was happening to her. She sought out doctors who just said she was depressed and needed some rest. But Cohen knew in her heart that she was not suffering from depression. She refused to take the doctor's orders to begin a prescription for antidepressants—there must be another way. After hours of research and reading, Cohen decided to embark on a massage therapy course, believing healing the muscular body could mitigate the illness within. One of her classes disclosed a specific treatment called "rain drop therapy," which is an aromatherapy massage technique in which you apply undiluted essential oils to your skin (Monroe, 2017). Cohen was instantly enchanted by the power and range of therapeutic oils. According to Cohen, "From the very first moment with those oils, I noticed that something was firing that hadn't been firing. I was deeply moved (Monroe, 2017)."

The brain fog and mental fatigue that was previously present was gone. Now, Cohen has woven into her daily life an essential oil ritual. Every morning, she gently rubs frankincense into her scalp. When dealing with certain situations, such as battling an illness or working on an important project, she turns to her trusty essential oils to give her the strength and power she needs. Eucalyptus oil aids in fighting fever, while spearmint helps one focus and concentrate. The deeper her research went and the longer she practiced the application of essential oils, Cohen's life was transformed—so much so that she decided to dedicate her life to becoming an advocate for the oils and spreading the message of their power (Monroe, 2017).

Discovering Essential Oils

Today, essential oils are known not only for their strong fragrances, but also as an integral alternative medicine that provides healing, clarity, and calm for millions of people. Essential oils are distilled from plants and considered a chemical compound that is a volatile liquid. The intensity of these oils is the reason they are blended to create an aromatherapy oil, cream, balm, salt, or gel. Caution is encouraged with essential oils as they can be extremely strong and cause reactions. Aromatherapy blends essential oils with other natural oils to create a subtle scent and a gentler medicinal oil. The form and method of this integrative medicine harnesses the power of natural and organic plant extracts to uplift emotional and physical well-being. There are hundreds of essential oils, each promoting a different type of healing or uplifting benefit. For example, lavender is commonly used to treat insomnia, while sandalwood is applied to soothe anxious minds.

How were these essential oils discovered? Essential oils and their healing properties have been utilized and cherished for thousands of years. Essential oils were blended into balms and resins in ancient China, Egypt, and India while being integrated for both spiritual and medical purposes. In ancient Egypt, oils are believed to have been used in the early ages of 4,500 BC (Cronkleton, 2019). Authoritative figures would indulge in essential oils not only as a luxury but as a vehicle to transmute with the gods. High priests used essential oils in rituals, each specific fragrance aligned with different gods depending on their benefits. Vials of essential oils were also stored with mummies and the dead to help guide them through the hereafter and ensure that their resting souls were able to experience a sweet-smelling afterlife. Pharaohs harnessed the power of essential oils, often creating their own aromatherapy blend for specific purposes such as meditation or to enhance their strength for war.

However, essential oils were used in a more practical manner as well. The ancient Egyptians recognized the medicinal properties such as their anti-fungal and anti-inflammatory capabilities. In fact, essential oils were a crucial part of the embalming process and were required to preserve the body.

In ancient India, the traditional and sacred medicine known as Ayurveda utilized essential oils and infused them into elixirs and potions for ailments to bolster spiritual, emotional, and physical healing. It has been recorded that the ancient Indian medicinal and spiritual healers curated and incorporated over 700 types of essential oils in their practices. Even during the Bubonic plague, Ayurveda and its use of essential oils were proven to be more beneficial and effective than antibiotics, eventually replacing them altogether (Cronkleton, 2019).

Later on, the acclaimed civilizations of Rome and Greece would trade these oils in vast amounts across the continent. The essential oils became aromatherapy by infusing flowers, leaves, and fragrant roots with animal fat and then rubbed on the skin. Essential oils were seen as a sign of wealth and used mainly for cosmetic purposes, including deodorant, hair products, and incense within the home. (Noyes, 2015). The actual distilling process of the oils from plant matter was discovered in Persia in the 10th century, this became the basis and foundation to extract concentrated essential oils.

As essential oils continued to gain in popularity across the world in the Middle Ages, the technique of distillation spread and reached Europe and was quickly adopted by what was then seen as medieval pharmacies. Plants and their accommodating smells were used for all kinds of ailments, with more essential oils being discovered on a regular basis. This era gave rise to oils such as cedarwood, sage, cinnamon, geranium, and rose. Once trade became possible popular, essential oils became one of the prominent trading foundations between European and the Asian countries. The essence of plants were fervently shared among foreign lands. This was the spark that kickstarted a legendary revolution of holistic healing with aromatherapy.

Finally, in modern times—more specifically the 19th century— essential oils were proven to have outstanding medicine properties. Lavender oil was one of the first oils to be recognized as a holistic, natural, and organic healer. Today, research is constantly being undertaken to further validate the extent of healing properties essential oils contain. In the 21st century the continued the use and importance attributed to aromatherapy which is now recognized as aroma science therapy (Ali, et al., 2015). Utilized for thousands of years, spanning from some of the most ancient civilizations to the most modern societies essential oils clearly have a positive impact, and they are here to stay. Let's find out more of the scientific aspect of essential oils that we use every day.

The Science Behind Aromatherapy

The actual organic, natural plant oil can be found in various areas of a plant, including the hairs and cells. The plants oils or essence shields the plant against bacteria and fungi. The aroma molecules within the essence are completely free from disease and infection, making them attractive elements to fight infections in the human body. In fact, the makeup of plant essence and oils are extremely similar to the form of human hormones, further proving their effectiveness for use in the human body.

When you inhale the scent of an essential oil the odor molecules stimulate thousands of olfactory membrane receptors as they travel through the nose. These molecules may journey to the lungs through the respiratory system or to various parts of the brain, such as the limbic region. Some oils generate signals that ignite the release of endorphins, which then travels to the nervous system and causes the entire body to relax and feel a sense of pleasure.

Essential oils are known and proven to have a wide variety of benefits, both medicinally and psychologically. Peppermint oil is commonly used to treat migraines and headaches. Inhaling lavender oil before going to bed can often help mitigate insomnia, especially in women after childbirth. Lavender or rose have been reported to reduce side effects for those going through cancer treatments. A combination of thyme and oregano essential oils are known to gently reduce inflammation. Tea tree oil is particularly popular ingredient when creating an antimicrobial or antibacterial blend.

Many have found aromatherapy is used, acclaimed, and cherished as elixirs for those suffering from anxiety and stress. In a recent study, the application and smell of rose geranium and rose water were proven to reduce levels of stress in patients, to a dramatic effect. Other oils commonly used to treat those suffering from anxiety include lavender, lemon, and bergamot essential oils (Barati et al., 2016).

A study was performed and reported in Nephro-Urology Monthly on the effects of using lavender and rose essential oils on 130 students (Barati et al., 2016). They were to inhale a lavender and rose oil blend for half an hour every night before bed. After four weeks of following the program, the student's anxiety levels were tested again. The results showed a dramatic reduction in anxiety levels. Many studies of a similar sort have been conducted and concluded similar results (Barati et al., 2016).

One of the most revealing studies was performed in 2014 by Shuk Kwan Tang and M. Y. Mimi Tse from the "Department of Orthopaedics & Traumatology" in the United Christian Hospital, and the School of Nursing in the Hong Kong Polytechnic University respectively. In this research program, 82 patients over 65 years of age were included, of which 44 were placed into the aromatherapy group and given a mixture of lavender and bergamot essential oils (Tang & Tse, 2014).

First, they were taught what aromatherapy was and how it worked and were given a customized four-week program to follow. This included four sessions, once a week, with an aromatherapist and a ritual to follow when at home for self-administration. An assessment of each patient's stress, pain, and anxiety levels was conducted. It was concluded that every single participant had suffered from chronic pain and anxiety for over three months. The levels of stress and frequency of pain differed, displaying the variety of problems found within the group of patients (Tang & Tse, 2014).

After the four-week program, the controlled group of 44 elderly participants all recorded that their anxiety and pain levels dropped dramatically. Every single one of them also concluded that they no longer required pharmaceuticals but instead relied on balms and oils to soothe their physical and mental pains and ailments. The study concluded that essential oils and aromatherapy are indeed extremely effective when it comes to treating and mitigating pain, both on a physical level and an emotional one (Tang & Tse, 2014).

The research program further concluded that the inhalation of essential oils, especially lavender and bergamot, are effective antidepressants and natural anxiety remedies. When one inhales essential oils, it's absorbed and transported through the olfactory pathway and then into the brain. These pleasant aromas uplift emotions and create a more peaceful environment, one that promotes a sense of calm and clarity (Tang & Tse, 2014).

Using Aromatherapy For Wellness

Before beginning your journey of aromatherapy, it is recommended you meet with an aromatherapist. It is beneficial for you to be aware of what your issues are, the more details you can provide the more applicable the recommendation can be. Start working with an aromatherapy specialist to choose the oils and techniques that will best suit your wellness needs.

There are hundreds of types of essential oils, each hold properties that are beneficial for distinctive issues, such as to soothe stress or help cultivate a more focused mind. There are two major groups that every essential oil falls under: nervine or sedative. The nervine group is attributed to the essential oils that strengthen the nervous system, while the sedative group calms and soothes the nervous system.

Aromatherapy can be used in a diffuser that slowly heats the oil to release a fragrant scent. The inhalation of essential oils can have direct and immediate beneficial and positive effects on your limbic system— the region of the brain that plays a crucial role in processing emotions and long-term memory retention. Most importantly, the limbic system is responsible for monitoring and controlling our unconscious actions, such as our heartbeat, breathing, blinking, and blood pressure regulation. Which are often areas where our anxiety manifests. Having a tool that can be helpful to manage reactions in this part of our body a healthy healing option.

Remember essential oils are often extremely potent, creating an aromatherapy blend makes it easier for the body to absorb this holistic medicine. Below is a list of some essential oils, their properties, and what they can be used for in relations to anxiety, depression, difficulty sleeping, and more (Cuncic, 2020; organicfact.net, healthline.com; naturallivingfamily.com; healthline.com)

- **Basil**: This cooking herb provides relief for nervous tension, migraines, and mental fatigue. It often acts as an antidepressant as well as helping soothe any panic attacks. Sweet Basil has studies showing instances of calming yet also, stimulating and uplifting the mind.

- **Bergamot**: The citrus, spicy scent of this plant attracts attention as studies show it improves moods and relieves anxiety. It regularly reduces inflammation, increasing positive mood, and there are reports it lowers cholesterol levels.

- **Chamomile**: This plant when used offers antioxidants to assist with sleep. It is ideal to reduce nausea and to soothe the nervous system, helpful for anxiety and depression.

- **Clary Sage**: This plant with purple tinted leaves is used as a sedative, relieving nervous tension. The smell of this ancient herb generates a sense of wellbeing, as it reduces feelings of anxiety. Stories indicate it has a history of healing wounds.

- **Clove**: These dried flower buds are not only healthy for gums and also relieves tooth pain, because of their antibacterial and anti-fungal attributes.

- **Eucalyptus:** This type of plant is known for opening the airways, reducing coughs, controlling blood sugar, and freshening breath. It frequently enhances feelings of relaxation as it reduces nervous tension.

- **Frankincense**: This oil has a long history and is known for anti-bacterial, anti-septic, and anti-inflammatory attributes. Promising indicators show it may improve asthma, arthritis, gut issues, and reduce cancer.

- **Geranium**: An oil with sedative properties that show a reduction of feeling stressed and anxious.

- **Jasmine**: This floral scent is both sweet and exotic. People report feeling calm, relaxed, and content after use. Reported to decrease depression and raise self-esteem.

- **Lavender**: This plant and flower are incredibly influential if you desire to calm the mind or to induce sleep. It also offers antibacterial properties.

- **Lemon**: This tangy fruit is an amazing disinfectant. Its attributes include anti-inflammatory and anti-microbial aspects that can reduce stress, elevate one's mood, and mental clarity.

- **Mandarin**: This citrus oil is a sedative that often relaxes and calms nervous issues while dissipating tension and anxiety.

- **Marjoram**: A traditional herb used to reduced nervousness and reports state it relieves headaches.

- **Peppermint**: This plant is known to kill germs, reduce itching, calm upset stomach, and increase blood circulation.

- **Rose**: This flower is a powerful stress, anxiety, and depression reliever. Reports indicate it has been known to assist in fading scars.

- **Sandalwood**: This bark has calming abilities that help ease anxiety, depression, and hypertension. At times it is used as an anti-viral antiseptic.

- **Valerian Root**: An ancient plant whose original use was to calm nerves making it easier to sleep. Known to reduce anxiety.

- **Ylang Ylang**: A flower who's oil can be used as a natural, non-steroidal, anti-inflammatory insect repellent and lower blood pressure for some.

Besides having strong fragrances which can be used as a perfume, essential oils can be used in many different ways. Again we want to stress if you are not familiar with essential oils, you will be using them as medicine so start by working with a knowledgeable aromatherapist. This person is educated in knowing how much to blend or dilute an essential oil for effectiveness and safety. Here are some techniques for you to consider:

- Inhale the scent, apply a drop or two to your palms or wrists, after diluting the essential oil. Use a cotton ball or piece of fabric, apply a few drops and hold it toward your nose, then inhale.

- Steam your face. All you need is a bowl, a towel, boiling water, and the essential oil you choose. Put boiling water in a bowl, apply two or three drops to your water, place the towel over your head and bowl so little air can get through, and breathe in the scented steam. If desired additional drops of oil can be added in small quantities.

- Diffuser, this can be a simple structure with a dish to hold water and essential oil while space below allows for a tea candle. When the candle has been lit, it slowly heats up the oil, which then evaporates and lets off the scent. There are also electric diffusers which also couple up as dehumidifiers to ensure stable and healthy air quality as well as applying a sweet or healing scent into the room.

- Cotton ball or fabric, apply a few drops place it next to your night table to inhale a calming oil to assist in getting to sleep and staying asleep.

- Create a balm, cream, gel, or blended oil, with an essential oil, then you can safely use this plant medicine on your skin. You simply need to identify the spot you wish to relax and gently rub your solution into that point, joint, or muscle. (When applying oil onto your skin, work with an aromatherapy expert and be aware of how potent the essential oil is.)

- Add to your shower. Eucalyptus is a popular shower essential oil as it is beneficial for breathing and the lungs. A result of both the humidity and heat within the shower, you will be able to experience the full benefits of the oils.

- Include a few drops to your bath for another way to use your essential oil. The essential oil will then be absorbed by the skin and soothe your muscles and mind. Add a few drops to your soap or bath salts.

- Create an aromatic room spray. In your home, you can combine some essential oil drops with water and mix them together in a spray bottle.

- Experience an overall affect, if you do not have a specific pain point, gently rub a calming aromatherapy lotion onto your temples, behind the ears, or your third eye.

Essential oils can be extremely beneficial on a physical, mental, emotional, and spiritual, level. With a wide range of scents and methods to incorporate them into daily life, it's no wonder these seemingly miraculous elixirs were used thousands of years ago and impressively are widely popular today. Using aromatherapy that is best for you can provide a soothing and relaxing impact. By simply breathing you can reduce tension and irritability.

Reflection

Be honest if you have an allergy to scents, there are other options to consider? Is aromatherapy a tool you would like to consider?

- Do you have the freedom to consider aromatherapy?

- Where will you look for and find an aromatherapy specialist near you?

- Which of the many techniques listed above would be easy to integrate into your life?

- How often might you use those techniques?

- Which essential oils are being recommended by a specialist?

- Decide how you will measure the impact.

Notes & things to remember....

CHAPTER THREE

━ ∷ ━

TAPPING RELEASES ANXIETY

Tapping is a modality that focuses on the senses of hearing and touching. This is a proven modality that you customize for yourself, it utilizes your energy that flows through acupuncture meridians. There are numerous tapping techniques we will introduce you to three and go in depth into Emotional Freedom Tapping (EFT). All are legitimate and are worth considering. Our story shares how a child with anxiety benefited from tapping. Also included is a tapping example for anxiety, and a question to decide if this technique would be useful medicine for your anxiety toolbox.

A Story About Tapping

Danielle's son was having trouble at school. As a result, he had trouble sleeping. But it was the rise of the virus and the harsh turn of events and transformation of life that set him off the most, and he eventually developed insomnia. He began panicking about the state of the world and worried constantly about his friends and loved ones who he could no longer see. Danielle knew she had to do something to help ease his suffering, soothe his nervous system, and calm his mind. So, she decided to turn to Emotional Freedom Tapping, more commonly referred to as EFT (Ortner, 2020).

Before bed, when Danielle's son's anxiety began to escalate yet again, she would ask him to say this mantra. "Even though I am feeling all this anxiety that is keeping me from sleeping, I deeply love and accept myself," and repeat it a handful of times. They would then proceed to their tapping exercise, gently touching certain points of the body to induce a sense of muscle relaxation that additional transference to the mind. Soon, she would notice her son's face relax, his eyes dropping, and then he'd let out a giant yawn. It was time for bed (Ortner, 2020).

However, it wasn't enough for a long-term solution. One day, Danielle walked into her son having a full-blown anxiety attack. His anxiety about the state of the world had become too much for his young mind, and he could no longer handle the immense stressful burden that weighed on his small shoulders. Danielle knew EFT was effective with some form of anxiety but had never used it to treat an intense anxiety attack before. She had nothing to lose and decided to try it out of desperation for the situation; she went through the tapping exercises with her son.

Within a mere 10 minutes, Danielle's son had calmed down. His heart rate decreased, and his breathing turned to normal. He had come back to her. He was in control of his body again. To this day, Danielle praises EFT and highly recommends it to anyone suffering from anxiety, whether it be mild or too much to bear (Ortner, 2020).

Tapping Therapy Overview

Life is filled with circumstances and situations that can induce anxiety. Stress is woven into the very fabric of reality, existence, and the human experience most days. However, there are many external properties that can bring forth unnecessary anxiety, which is harmful to our bodies and minds. For example, the novel coronavirus has not only brought a physical disease into the midst of the world, but it also crept into the crevices of every society, city, and home. In response to this widespread, global pandemic everyone is experiencing an increased level of anxiety.

There are three well known tapping modalities that incorporate tapping to help with anxiety and emotional wellbeing:

- Thought Field Therapy (TFT) founded in 1980 by Roger Callahan

- Tapas Acupressure Therapy (TAT) founded by Tapas Fleming in 1993

- Emotional Freedom Technique (EFT) which originated in 1995 by Gary Craig

Each tapping techniques has distinctive styles and philosophies. All of them focus on keeping energy flowing through your energy meridians to keep your body healthy. EFT is a powerful technique used to soothe, halt, and release anxiety and stress, as well as, weight gain, self-esteem issues, and productivity, to name a few. Tapping is an effective tool to mitigate common problems that have endured since ancient times and continue to be with us in modern day.

Acupuncture, a treatment technique within Traditional Chinese Medicine (TCM), believes meridians keep energy flowing in our bodies. This energy is referred to as "chi" or "qi", which constantly moves along 12 major meridians that are pathways throughout the body, each intercept our various organs. There are additional meridians, but we will not go into depth on those. Meridians do not exist physically as they are energetic paths that keep chi circulating, so our bodies can function at our highest level of health and wellness. When meridians are open and channeling energy it generates calm, clarity, and balance in our bodies. Tapping techniques accept this energetic philosophy and stimulate various points of the meridians to generate results.

The Science Behind Tapping Therapy

Stress, anxiety, or fear stimulate the amygdala, a complex group of brain cells in the center of the brain, that is known for processing emotions and memories related to fear. The amygdala notifies the nervous system and your innate response to fear is set in motion. This automatic response causes the adrenal glands to produce adrenaline and cortisol. Today, we may have racing minds or face triggers that are overwhelming and initiate panic attacks, Understanding triggers and how your body is responding is integral for you to choose which alternative approach offers the best solution. Generally, tapping helps our brains calm down and halts the release of these hormones. This gives you the ability to take a step back and view your situation in a calmer way.

Tapping EFT points, aligned with the meridians used in acupuncture, informs your body that you are not in danger. When we pair a mantra with our tapping exercises, we further wire our brain to feel peaceful. A mantra can be simple. For example, you can repeat the phrase, "I am safe;

I am supported; I am loved" while tapping your main EFT points and focusing on your current emotions and feelings. Tapping and speaking the mantra inform the brain that the body is in a space to relax and release tension. It almost instantly brings clarity to the mind and eases thoughts of anxiety.

Dr. Peta Stapleton from Bond University in Australia conducted a research program on tapping in 2020 (Mackintosh & Stapleton, 2020). She gathered 53 patients and randomly placed them in groups of three. One group was to do nothing, the second group was asked to read psychology books, and the third group was assigned a tapping technique. Each group was to perform their task for a period of 60 minutes. Before the research began, Stapleton tested every participant's cortisol levels—the hormone that indicates stress and anxiety. After an hour of either sitting, reading, or going through the tapping method, Stapleton then tested each member's cortisol levels. While there were no significant drops of cortisol levels in the first two groups, the tapping group results stated that an average of a 43% decline in cortisol levels was found. In just an hour, basically every group participant had relaxed by nearly 50% (Mackintosh & Stapleton, 2020). Demonstrating EFT has been found to significantly reduce anxiety and stress.

Tapping not only halts the release of these anxiety-inducing hormones but also regulates and soothes the nervous system. A reduction of cortisol also helps the body fight inflammation, while an increase of cortisol causes a rise in inflammation. Additionally, EFT bolsters the strength of the immune system by reverting the body back into a parasympathetic response, otherwise known as relaxation. When we are stressed, our body places nearly all of our energy and focus on the problem at hand. Fortunately, when we are relaxed, our body focuses its energy on building strength and health.

These can be the direct results of tapping but not the only ones. Creating a tapping routine and regularly practicing it on a daily level, you can regulate your cortisol levels to a suitable level for you. This can help both the mind and body in a multitude of ways. In the long run, you will be able to handle difficult situations more easily, you'll have increased self-awareness and confidence. You can also improve your sleeping patterns, which often reduces irritability, improving many aspects of your life. With tapping, you are equipped with a simple, yet incredibly effective, tool to battle negative energies or emotions that has been scientifically proven time and time again.

Make Tapping A Part Of Life

EFT is used to relieve feelings of stress and anxiety, it is easy to integrate into your everyday life. Once you get comfortable with the process you can use it to assist with getting to sleep or reversing anxiety before it escalates. This is a general description of what it it like working with a certified EFT practitioner. The patient is first asked to describe what is up for them at this moment, focusing on their emotions to identify the problem. Once the problem has been identified, the practitioner and patient create a mantra, and follow it with an unconditional affirmation. It is important to rate the intensity of the of the problem from 0-10 so the patient knows where they are beginning.

While placing deep attention on the feeling itself, the patient begins by repeating the statement 3 times while making karate chops on the outer part of the hands. This offers time to confirm the mantra feels right. Then progress to tapping with two fingertips between five and seven times on the specific meridian points while saying the mantra. There are numerous ways to explore and experience the benefits of tapping, here is one tapping sequence that remains both a basis and foundation in a more traditional sense, that may work its magic for you:

1. The karate chops are on the outer sides of your hands below the little fingers.

2. The top of your head in the center;

3. Between the eyebrows—where each brow begins where it connects with your nose;

4. Both outside corners of the eyes;

5. Under the center points of the eyes;

6. Underneath the nose;

7. The chin below the bottom lip;

8. An inch below the collarbone;

9. Either side of your body about four to five inches below the armpit;

10. Return to the top of head in the center.

Here is a more detailed description. First, begin observing and naming your emotion. Is it anger, anxiety, or stress, or tension? Once you have identified your issue, rate its intensity on a scale of zero to 10. It is important to create and repeat a mantra, or what is more commonly known to the tapping community as a setup statement. This can be a phrase that further vocalizes the troubling situation that overwhelms you, followed by a positive statement. For example, "I may be feeling extremely anxious, and I still support, accept, and love myself." Once the setup statement resonates, move through the tapping areas gently while repeating your mantra. Remember to start with the karate chop part on the side of your hands, then go to the crown of your head and move downward, through the remaining locations, ending the sequence by returning to tap the top of the head again. Rate the intensity of the issue to clarify the impact of the tapping sequence. If the issue persists, perform another round of tapping. When you are new continue to use the same setup statement, as you get more comfortable with the process you can change the mantra slightly at each tapping point.

This is the only technique in this book where following examples on YouTube are useful, as you can see the actual areas to tap. For examples you can watch the following videos, or others, on YouTube:

- Nick Ortner's Tapping Technique to Calm Anxiety & Stress in 3 Minutes (Nick Ortner's Tapping Technique to Calm Anxiety & Stress in 3 Minutes, 2020)

- How to Tap with Jessica Ortner: Emotional Freedom Technique Informational Video (How to Tap with Jessica Ortner: Emotional Freedom Technique Informational Video, 2013)

- How TAPPING Can Help Reduce Stress & Anxiety About Coronavirus (How TAPPING Can Help Reduce Stress & Anxiety About Coronavirus, 2020)

Here is a thorough example that you can personalize so it is aligned with your concerns and becomes comfortable for you. To see if there is a change, take a minute to rate from 0-10: your level of anxiety; your level of stress; rate one part of your body that holds your tension; what is the level of your racing mind?

Below are potential first round setup statements for a tapping exercise concerned with anxiety, you can follow the first phrase while you move through each motion. To begin with, choose one phrase and repeat it throughout the process.

1. Start by repeating the setup statement 3 times while making karate chops on the outer part of your hands.

2. Tap the crown of your head and say out loud: "This anxiety (fill in the blank). . ."

3. Tap the center eyebrow region and say: "All of this anxiety about (fill in the blank) . . ."

4. Tap on the outer side of the eyes and repeat: "All this stress about (fill in the blank) . . ."

5. Tap underneath the center point of the eyes and say, ". . . (fill in the blank) is exhausting."

6. Tap underneath the nose and say out loud: "All of this stress (fill in the blank). . ."

7. Tap beneath the bottom lip on the chin center and repeat: "All this anxiety (fill in the blank) . . ."

8. Tap beneath both collar bones and say: "I'm feeling anxious (fill in the blank). . ."

9. Tap underneath the armpits and repeat: "and I don't know what to do about it."

10. Return to Tap the crown of your head and say out loud ......

Take two deep breaths in and out. Pause. Look at the issues you rated prior to tapping and write down the intensity of the issues. Compare with the original ratings to see for yourself if there is a positive change. If needed complete a second round.

Here are potential second round mantras to consider:

1. Start by repeating the setup statement 3 times while making karate chops on the outer part of your hands.

2. Tap the crown of your head and say out loud: "This anxiety (fill in the blank). . ."

3. Tap the center eyebrow region and say: "All of this worrying (fill in the blank). . .

4. Tap on the outer side of the eyes and repeat: "All this stress about (fill in the blank) . . ."

5. Tap underneath the center point of the eyes and say: "This issue of . . . (fill in the blank) . . ."

6. Tap underneath the nose and say out loud: This issue (fillin the blank) . . ."

7. Tap beneath the bottom lip on the chin center and repeat: "...
   is causing me discomfort."

8. Tap beneath both collar bones and say: "All of this fear ..."

9. Tap underneath the armpits and repeat: "... is too much ..."

10. Return to Tap the crown of your head and say out loud: "... but
    I choose to love and accept myself no matter what."

Take two deep breaths in and out. Pause. Rate the intensity of your
anxiety; your level of stress; your racing mind; rate the part of your
body you chose, to specify the impact of the tapping. By now, your
cortisol levels have dropped slightly. If you're still feeling overwhelmed or
anxious, continue with another round. One to four rounds are usually
effective for many people, but if you're still rating your intensity of
emotions on the higher level of the scale, you can repeat the process and
rounds a few more times. Filled with a sense of love and acceptance,
paired with the tapping that is sending calming signals to the brain,
you will be able to relax, release tension, and begin clearing the mind's
overwhelming feeling.

EFT holds numerous benefits. Tapping is incredibly good for sedating
stress and emotions stemming from anxiety. As mentioned previously,
tapping can have a positive impact on the region of the brain that
tackles the fight-or-flight response, otherwise known as survival mode
instincts. This area releases stress hormones. When a patient utilizes
tapping, it sends relaxing signals to the brain and halts the release of these
hormones.

The gift of EFT is as its name suggests—freedom from the negative emotions, stress, tension, and irritability that are limiting the joy in your life. Tapping has been researched to show the benefits people experience by personalizing this process. This technique is self-driven with setup statements you customize to acknowledge where you are and give yourself inspiration to move forward to a healthier place. You know yourself best. If anyone can describe your pain and know what inspires you – it's YOU. Try tapping when you are triggered and see if you breathe easier, regain your control, and calm yourself from within using this incredibly soothing practice.

Reflection

Consider tapping for ease and relief.

- Does Tapping feel comfortable for you to use?

- What situations does tapping give you the strength to take charge of your anxiety?

- Will you invite someone to tap with you or practice alone?

- Where will you look for videos that show the tapping locations?

- How will you measure the benefits of tapping?

Notes & Things to remember:

Chapter Four

— . —

Exercise As Medicine For Anxiety

For almost every ailment one of the top three ways to shift onto a healthier track is exercise. Movement can be medicine, 100% applicable for anxiety and may offer positive side effects for your concentration loss, lack of sleep, muscle tension, and racing mind. Exercise is another very easy to integrate modality that can begin at any level. If you have not been consciously moving throughout your day make sure to consult your doctor first. This complementary approach is kinesthetic and works with the senses of seeing, hearing, and touching. In this chapter you will learn how others with anxiety benefited from exercise, a variety of exercise styles to choose from, and a potential structure to integrate it for a healthier life.

A Story - The Impact Of Movement

Charlotte Anderson felt like a prisoner to her anxiety. It controlled her every thought, emotion, and action. She became too much of a slave to her stress that she didn't leave her house in an entire year. Then, she received an invite to her sister's wedding. She couldn't miss it. She had to do something; she had to break free somehow. She no longer wanted to be a fearful person missing out on all the joys of life because her overthinking mind held her at bay. Anderson went to see her doctor, and she was given a hard pill to swallow: the truth. She was a pre-type 2 diabetic, overweight, and her physical issues were constantly fueling her emotional responses to everything, causing panic attacks and regular gusts of stress and anxiety. She was sick. She was unhappy (Anderson, 2016).

It took her a while, but Anderson delved deep to find the courage to begin her healing journey. She made a promise to herself to lose weight for health reasons. She started creating awareness around her eating habits, noticing that her stress sparked a need for unhealthy comfort foods. Anderson started changing her eating habits. Then, she decided to start walking. First, 20 minutes around the block, then a bit farther for 30 minutes. After she grew used to her walking, she started jogging. Six months after her health epiphany and renewal, she was running five times a week, embarking on various fitness journeys, lifting weights, and taking part in high-intensity interval training (HIIT). As her weight dropped and health increased, her confidence grew. Her self-esteem started to shine. After a year, she was competing in half marathons (Anderson, 2016).

Over three years later, Anderson is in an incredibly fit state, both mentally and physically. She is no longer pre-diabetic and she has restored her strength—so much so that she no longer has anxiety. Her confidence and power have crushed the forces that held her back. Anderson broke free of her mental imprisonment. Fitness and exercise saved her life (Anderson, 2016).

Exercise Therapy Overview

Though this is only one example, it shows that exercise has seemingly endless benefits to both the body and mind, which often then uplift spirit. Physical movement is an incredibly powerful tool to mitigate, halt, and even reverse the negative effects of anxiety, with the possibility of eradicating anxiety. It is one of the most basic and simplest modalities you can integrate into your everyday life, and it is never too late to begin. Exercise is a complementary approach. It stimulates nearly all of your senses: seeing, hearing, touching and smelling (breathing). The side effects often reconnect the body, balance the mind, and support overall health and well-being.

Our bodies are the vehicle from which we experience the world around us. Our ancestors, as well as every other being on this planet, continuously moved around. However, on a more specific level, the original homo sapiens needed to move around to find food, shelter, water, learn about their intimate surroundings, and environment. They had to sprint to catch prey, run away from potential dangers and predators, walk long distances to find a suitable food to gather, or move to a new living space. Movement is therefore an innate part of human lives.

In 3,000 and 1,000 BC, ancient Chinese medicine and wellness concepts outlined that exercise, such as Tai Chi and QiGong, were deeply connected to creating a balanced life that was in harmony with nature and the body. India followed with breathing and yoga, aspects of Ayurveda, which will be expanded upon in the next chapter. Thousands of years ago this collection of health and wellness ideals confirmed the dire need for movement in one's life. However, with the rise of the industrial revolution, humans began repetitive motions and no longer needed to move around as much. We never lost the knowledge and innate sense that being active was one of the most significant foundations in creating a healthy and long-lasting life.

Ancient civilizations, such as Egypt, Rome, and Greece, promoted exercise as one of the most divine activities and ways of life. War required strenuous movement and strength, the military took priority, and a healthy life was idealized as pure and unwavering beauty. Philosophy outlines exercise as one of life's most significant concepts to happiness. As humans evolved and society continued to develop, so did the various forms of exercise. Athletic ordeals and competitions even rose, thus the inception of the Olympic Games. Physical exercise began being taught in schools. However, in the 20th century exercise took a capitalistic and competitive direction. Fitness centers and gyms grew in popularity and more research was conducted to enhance physical activities and health. As science evolved, so did the understanding of how exercise impacts us. A sound body leads to a sound mind, which leads to a happy life.

In order to create a healthy, well-balanced, and resilient life, movement needs to be a part of your routine in some way. Whether it's a daily chair exercise, run, lifting weights, yoga in the mornings, or simply a stroll in a park, physical activity is one of the most important ingredients when it comes to inspiring enhanced well-being and happiness. Today, human beings still have our ancestors' bodies. These vessels ultimately require movement just as our ancestors performed daily tasks. In particular, exercise holds so many benefits when it comes to fighting stress and anxiety. It improves self-confidence, enhances resilience, builds the feeling of accomplishment, and wards off negative emotions.

Exercise doesn't have to be a chore, it doesn't have to be performed in a gym with expensive and complex equipment, and it definitely doesn't have to be strenuous. It's proven that even the simplest of physical movements can have great benefits on the mind and body.

Proven Benefits for Anxiety

Exercise can make you feel happier—it's proven. When we exercise, whether we're walking, running, swimming, cycling, or moving, our brain activates neurotransmitters such as Endorphins, then a cocktail of positive chemicals are released serotonin, dopamine, and norepinephrine. These chemicals allow us to feel a sense of calm and pleasure. As we invite exercise into our weekly or daily routines. Receiving regular hits of these pleasure-producing chemicals, our brain can rewire to fully accommodate this feeling, helping us alleviate stress, anxiety, and depression. Surprisingly, it doesn't actually matter how intense or calm your level of exercise is in order to release these chemicals and hormones. Even a simple stretch can have a positive impact.

How does exercise affect anxiety in a positive manner?

- Exercise gives your seemingly endless racing mind a rest by diverting your attention onto something else.

- Movement relieves muscle tension and soothes the nervous system, which is responsible for the physical effects of anxiety.

- Increasing your heart rate alters the chemistry of your brain, therefore increasing the release and transport of pleasure-producing neurochemicals, including serotonin.

In turn, the more energy you exude when exercising, the more energy you will build. You can adopt a renewed thirst for life, a longing to experience more, and refill your energetic chalice. Many of those who suffer from anxiety, stress, and depression have significantly decreased energy levels and also battle constant fatigue. However, regular exercise can combat this disillusionment and aid in alleviating anxiety. While these are mostly physical attributes that, in turn, affect the mental parts of human existence, exercise has a positive affect the brain. When you begin exercising, your heart rate increases due to the exertion of energy. The rate depends on the level of intensity and your personal fitness level. Regardless, when your heart rate increases, it improves and enhances the blood and oxygen flow to both the body and brain. This can actually trigger the brain's production of specific hormones that help grow and strengthen brain cells. Over time, you can develop a stronger sense of mental clarity, focus, and memory.

Physical movement also aids in better sleeping patterns and relaxation. When you expel energy during exercise, the body tends to be more relaxed as it is no longer holding on to tension. This often makes it easier to sleep, allowing your body the down time used for your daily recuperation process. Additionally, sleep allows your subconscious space to process the day and allowing your mind to take a break from stressful emotions. All factors that impact the ability to concentrate, calm a racing mind and manage anxiety. Consider this alternative to boost your strength, soothe your mind, and act as a powerful tool to alleviate anxiety.

Create A Movement Routine

In terms of anxiety, choose what works best for you, given where you are. Consult a doctor if you are uncertain. A 10-minute walk could have the same benefits on the mind as a 45-minute jog. Be mindful while you take on your physical exercise. Be grateful for the fact that you have a body you can move and that you have the time and are using it to better yourself. As you push past all your mental obstacles you will not only achieve physical fitness but mental and emotional strength. You'll be more adept to handle stressful situations while bolstering your immune system and overall health. You'll be more open to fresh perspectives, new experiences, and even reach new heights, both metaphorically and literally.

Our minds are more powerful than our bodies and often, we can talk ourselves out of things that are good for us. The first thing we recommend doing, in order to incorporate exercise into your everyday life, is shift your mindset, get an exercise buddy, ask for a friend to encourage you daily, or make a commitment to a class.

Here are a few supportive steps you can take:

- **Set an intention**.

- **Describe how you want to feel**... How would you explain feeling relieved? How would a calmer mind change your day?

- **Start small and build momentum**.

- **Let go of thinking about exercise as an all-or-nothing** concept. Don't let yourself ponder on having to perform strenuous physical activities to gain anything. Perhaps begin with a 15 or 20-minute walk. Consider stretching before going to bed. Every little bit truly does count and makes a difference.

- Find an exercise that you enjoy and **be patient with yourself, consistency is key**. Don't aim too high too quickly. As the popular phrase goes, Rome wasn't built in a day, and good things take time. Don't expect your life to change overnight.

- **Find a buddy or two**, the more the merrier and the higher the probability you will motivate each other to stay active. Pair up with a friend or create a fitness group. Hold each other accountable, get social, and then treat yourselves to a healthy beverage after your amazing workout.

As time progresses evaluate the impact of the exercise on your body, energy, and mental state. Set desired milestones and rate where you are in the beginning, how your are progressing, as well as where you want to advance. Doing exercise is valuable, becoming who you want can be magical.

Here are some tricks to create time to exercise during your day: Incorporate movement into your to-do list; wake up a 15-30 minutes earlier; listen to your favorite music or an interesting podcast while performing your exercise; learn something while you are moving or make the activity fun; add some dance moves into your daily chores; take the stairs; park further away from the entrance so you take extra steps; do some jumping jacks while you wait for your bath to fill. Believe in your promise to yourself, you are worth it.

There are hundreds of exercise types, but some are particularly effective when it comes to fighting, alleviating, and reducing anxiety and feelings of stress.

- Aerobic exercises are the forms of movement to best increase your heart rate so you can receive the maximum results plus benefits that soothe stress and anxiety. These include swimming, cycling, running, dancing, hiking, boxing, and tennis.

- Yoga is incredibly calming and effective for both the mind and body; it works cooperatively to shift emotional states. If you have physical limitations, consider starting with chair yoga.

- Breathing exercises offer an incredible healthy approach that instantly quiets the nervous system, expands your lung capacity, helps you reconnect to your center, by connecting to your breath.

- It is highly recommended for humans to spend time in nature.

Many of us live in cities, so we often find ourselves disconnected from nature, which can aggravate our anxious minds. Spending time in nature can calm us and put our minds at ease. Another joyful exercise option is gardening, it requires an increased amount of movement as you get up and down and can offer you similar benefits as other forms of exercise. A connection to the Earth and spending time outdoors thus positively impacts and improves your quality of life.

Given there are so many types of exercise, and everyone is at a different level, here are a few lists we hope you will find to be a useful resource:

- 101 Bodyweight Exercises That You Can Do Anywhere
  https://travelstrong.net/bodyweight-exercises/

- The Ultimate List of Compound
  Exercises: 50 Muscle-Building Exercises
  https://thefitnesstribe.com/list-of-compound-exercises/

- 30 Moves to Make the Most of Your At-Home Workout (all
  levels)
  https://www.healthline.com/health/fitness-exercise/at-home-
  workouts

- How to Start Working Out If You've Never Exercised Before
  https://www.self.com/story/steps-to-take-start-working-out-f
  or-first-time

Physical exercise has unlimited benefits on the mind and body. In particular, movement can be medicine and therapy for those suffering from anxiety, stress, and depression. It can alleviate the sensation of being overwhelmed and on edge by reducing the chemicals that trigger those emotions and feelings while releasing the hormones that instill a sense of pleasure within. If done on a regular basis and maintained consistently, these feelings of achievement and happiness can rewire the brain itself to search for the joy in everyday life, therefore making you more prone to happiness and more likely to ward off anxious, irritating thoughts. Exercise is one of the most powerful yet simple tools we can use to alleviate the stresses in our minds.

Reflection

Logically, we know, some form of movement is advantageous for us all. Is this a tool that you want to use to reduce your anxiety, irritation, or tension all over?

- What's your Why? Your ultimate motivation?

- What exercises do you enjoy that can be helpful?

- Write down your desired results from exercising.

- How will you measure getting there?

- Write down your preferred method of movement.

- Get specific with length of time, days of the week, and which hours of the day.

- Who can be your exercise buddy?

Notes & things to remember....

CHAPTER FIVE

— : —

AYURVEDA HELPS ANXIETY

This chapter will present one of the oldest and most all-encompassing modalities that can shift your way of life. Ayurveda has many facets you can incorporate a few aspects or all depending on how extreme your ailments are, how healthy you want to be, and what lifestyle aspects you are willing to change. This approach to life is often an extreme change for westerners, however it is one of the most powerful for your entire being. All of the senses are stimulated by Ayurveda. Incorporating panchakarma treatments, herbal remedies, and eating philosophy, must be done with a certified practitioner. Meditation, yoga, breathing exercises and bathing can be done on your own. This chapter will present a story, some ancient history, science, and practices that introduce you to some of the aspects of Ayurveda.

A Story About Ayurveda

Crystal Hoshaw (2020) started feeling anxious when she was just a child. As pressures from society were already weighing her down. School, grades, and social expectations caused emotions of fear and stress in her everyday life. Her anxiety continued through her teenage years, seeping into her age as a young adult ages. She knew she couldn't live like this anymore. To combat her seemingly unwavering anxiety, Crystal turned to one facet of Ayurveda, yoga. However, she still couldn't seem to shake her forever racing mind, with one imaginary problem to the next constantly popping into her head. Then, she learned more about Ayurveda and changed her life. She realized through the knowledge and lessons of this ancient, traditional, holistic Ayurveda medicine, from India, what she really needed to do was expand her perception and outlook on life. The way she approached every aspect and find a deep connection with her mind, body, and soul. Through detoxification methods, herbology, healthy consumption, cosmology, yoga, meditation, and mindfulness, Hoshaw was able to heal herself from her seemingly endless mental pains.

Today, Hoshaw is a yoga practitioner and anxiety healer. She found her strength from within, by embracing and loving helping hand of Ayurveda. She hasn't suffered from anxiety in years, and now, she helps others alleviate theirs (Hoshaw, 2020).

Ayurveda Overview

Ayurveda is a medical philosophy originating in India, that can also be an integrated approach to life. An Ayurveda doctor is referred to as a

Vaidya. The Ayurvedic Doctor's assistant is referred to as a Paricharaka, and an Ayurvedic Health Coach is often called Svastha Acharya. This integrative modality involves ancient assessment techniques, as well as the incorporation of herbs, treatments, cosmology, movement, breathing, mantras, energy flow through chakras, and diet. It's about reconnecting with the feelings of the body, truly listening, and responding to what the body is trying to tell us and understanding our relationship with the environment around us. Its foundation is based on the concept that every bodily element is connected. Diseases and illness, whether physical or mental, appear when the mind, body, heart, or spirit is out of harmony and balance. Ayurveda strives to balance mind, body, and spirit, to reduce stress and anxiety without any harm to nature or the person to uplift their well-being. This holistic lifestyle integrates: body and mind through yoga, meditation, mantras, and breathing; the senses of taste and smell through food and herbs; and treatments stimulate or calm the senses of seeing, hearing, and touching. It also follows the medicinal properties of plants as well as how senses interacts with the elements of the environment. It's designed to energize or calm your chakras. The desire is to help you understand and process life and how you interrelate to what surrounds you at the present moment.

The word Ayurveda takes its name from the Sanskrit language ayur, meaning life, and veda, which translates to knowledge or science, together it means the "knowledge of life." There is no way to respectfully describe Ayurveda in this introductory book. Here is a brief summary of its expansive concepts. The four Vedas compiled the knowledge, that explain the principles of the universe composed of five elements. This leads to three body variations referred to as Tridoshas. Balancing the natural elements and doshas in each body is the state of ultimate health. Where there is an imbalance there is illness or disease. The details and depth of this integrated approach to health is elaborate. Through the detoxification of impurities, the reduction of negative symptoms, the building of strength and resilience, and the decrease of stress and worrying, you can find a balanced, harmonious bliss within your life (Jaiswal & Williams, 2017).

Ayurveda originated around 3,000-6,000 years ago. It was conceived through the integration of the schools of ancient Hindu Philosophical teachings, Vaisheshika, and Nyaya, which preached pathological conditioning and logic respectively. However, many or all of those who practice and began the movement of Ayurveda hold the belief that it originated from divine intervention when the Hindu God Brahma, the creator of the entire universe, passed down holistic wisdom and knowledge of Earth and elements to the healing sages for the wellbeing of all. Whichever belief you choose, Ayurveda holds the pure knowledge of both plants and the earth, as well as the understanding of the human body, that forms these medical principles. As the system was enhanced, practiced, and developed, it grew in popularity. Its effectiveness further helped its use. The intricate and detailed methods were soon written in scripts in the Charak Samhita and Sushruta Samhita.

Ayurveda survived through centuries and was taught over generations due to its effectiveness of overcoming diseases throughout time. Therefore, families pass on healing traditions from previous generations, they don't always call it Ayurveda. Today, Ayurveda is still widely used in India, Nepal, Sri Lanka, Pakistan, Bangladesh and Myanmar, where it is seen as more valuable than Western medicine. There are institutions that train doctors and assistants, both these schools and healers are globally recognized. However, this form of medicine and healing is not commonly practiced or acclaimed in the United States of America but has been proven to have overall positive effects beyond what modern medicine can provide (Jaiswal & Williams, 2017).

Millions of people around the world have changed their lives with Ayurveda. It has not only aided them to overcome physical ailments but mental as well. It has uplifted the quality of lives and is known to be a powerful tool to soothe the anxious mind. The western approach to medicine provides a quick solution to symptoms, without identifying the source of illness. Ayurveda has an alternative approach that integrates the body, mind, and spirit to identify where the source of the imbalance is within the whole body. In terms of anxiety, stress, and depression, Ayurveda often proves to be far more effective than any Western medicine. However, that being said, it is still of vital importance that you consult an Ayurveda doctor or assistant before embarking on a healing journey such as this.

Ayurveda Principles And Beliefs

Knowing what little I do about Ayurveda, this will be a feeble attempt to give you an introduction to some of these honorable, ancient concepts. The beliefs begin with five primary elements that make up the universe and drive the energy forces within everything. This is air (vayu); water (jala); space / ether (aakash); earth (prithvi); and fire (teja), collectively the five elements are referred to as the Pancha Mahabhoota. They form a basis for three types of human bodies and their physiological functions, Tridoshas (Vata, Pitta, Kapha). When placing three earthly elements together, they maintain certain systems within the human body. The Vata Dosha regulates the excretion of waste products, the balance of electrolytes, and the transportation of cells. The Pitta Dosha maintains the thirst and pain management within the body's system, the body's temperature, and the coordination of the nerves. The Kapha Dosha provides the lubrication the body's joints required to function correctly.

One emphasis of Ayurveda's main treatments and principles is detoxification, there is discussion to evaluate waste produced by the body as it influences one's metabolism and digestion. When healthy, the body releases the oils and toxins that are no longer needed so you are able to reenergize, rejuvenate, and welcome what is actually meant for you to discover your higher form of energy and self. The physical toxins found within the body are the Tri Malas: the Mutra, the Purisa, and the Sveda, which are the urine, feces, and sweat respectively.

This ancient medical system further explains that if the waste products of the body are not released or maintained in a healthy way, numerous other factors will be affected in a negative way. It can cause a variety of other health issues physically and mentally. The Mutra needs to be excreted to avoid problems such as urinary tract infections, when not functioning properly the Sveda can cause skin problems, and an imbalance with the Purisa can cause constipation or diarrhea. In turn, these physical ailments can further cause mental issues such as anxiety and stress. An unbalanced physical system absolutely impacts your mental health. If you're feeling sick, you rarely feel happy and wholesome or fulfilled and uplifted. When you have a balanced and healthy system, you're regulating the correct functioning of your brain and hormones increasing concentration and reducing irritability (Jaiswal & Williams, 2017).

Another principle of Ayurveda also follows the biological fire that sits within us. This is our metabolic function, known as the Agni. There are 13 classifications that make up the entire agni and regulate the digestive system. The most important class is the Jatharagni, the fire within the digestive system itself. This flame is responsible for stimulating and regulating microflora, helping digestive functions, and supplying the entire body with energy. Anxiety is directly connected to the digestive tract and can cause serious harm to the microflora found within the digestive tract. This also affects the wellness of the mind, as the digestive tract helps regulate the transferal of hormones, such as cortisol, the hormone that produces feelings of anxiety. There are various therapeutic treatments called Panchakarma that are designed to detoxify the body, create a cleansing energy flow, release mental anxiety, and address all ailments.

According to Ayurveda, anxiety is considered to be an imbalance of the vata element of oneself—the air element. The air element imbalance often reveals sensations of overwhelm and may show up in the form of confusion, worrying, obsessing, overthinking, difficulty focusing, and at times trouble sleeping. This ungrounded feeling can mean that you have too much energy in your head and not enough in the physical body and especially your feet. One possibility recommended by Deepak Chopra on his website for healing anxiety is meditation "to stabilize your energy – calm the nervous system, relax the mind, release obsessive thoughts, connect to your body and to the earth."

All in all, to calm the mind both in the present and in the long run; to build up strength and resilience to the constant turmoil of life, you need to preserve and protect the physical and mental body. They work as one, with each and every component leaking and influencing one another. Look after your health, detox your body, and then look after your mind. If you attach a negative sensation to these words, counteract them with an action, experience, or behavior that you consider to be the opposite of the negative word, so there is no harm. Restore balance and harmony—revitalize your vata, or air flow, to soothe the mind.

Ayurveda Throughout Your Life

There are numerous ways to introduce Ayurveda techniques and practices into your life. These include: cultivating a meditation practice, nourishing yourself with food that aligns with your dosha, creating a sustainable daily routine that includes bathing (or showering), practicing yoga, visiting an Ayurveda doctor regularly to receive panchakarma treatments, and incorporating healthy herbs.

MEDITATION AND ANXIETY

Meditation is the act of finding peace and calm in the present moment through intentional focus. This concentration can be placed on the inhale and exhale of the breath, the sensations within the body, or on a mantra. Whatever the focal point may be, this ancient mindfulness practice is ideal to cultivate a sense of inner peace, even when your mind is racing or external circumstances may seem overwhelming.

The origin of meditation practice began as an ayurveda treatment and has expanded over the centuries to offer many contemporary options. Ultimately the intention is being able to experience awareness, harmony, inner calm, deep relaxation, and mindfulness. If you find meditation does not work for you it could be because it is not aligned with your mental constitution or mental state at that time. Ayurveda philosophy believes all is interrelated, so the status of your doshas, your health, your environment are all factors in your ability to integrate meditation into your life.

Each dosha responds best to a different type of meditation. Kapha is the walking meditation. Pitta is the pranayama or breathing meditation.

Vata is the mantra meditation. There are many forms of meditation that have evolved over time. To provide you options here are a variety of meditations, not limited to those sanctioned by Ayurveda philosophy.

- **Mindfulness** Meditation: This is the most popular form of meditative practice, particularly in Western civilizations. This is a simple session, where the mediator places their focus on their thoughts. However, rather than entertaining each thought, fleshing it out, and turning these patterns into a session of overthinking, the meditator must simply observe their thoughts and not attach any form or level of judgment to them. While you observe, you can also take note of your thinking, thought progressions, and patterns. This way, you can identify what it is that is troubling you currently in life, and what you might need to do to find inner peace. You can combine this practice with focusing on the breath, returning your concentration to the inhale and exhale when your thoughts start to prove overbearing.

- **Focused** Meditation: This is a meditation practice where you notice your five senses. Place your concentration on your breath, the smells around you, what you hear, the sensations against your skin, and what you taste. Then, choose one sense to place your focus on. Often, this practice can require tools to utilize such as prayer beads or the sound of a gong. This helps cultivate build concentration.

- **Spiritual** Meditation: This is a meditative session that honors and gives praise to the universe or a religious figure. It is often practiced in a place of worship and uses essential oils to heighten both the experience and the connection with a spiritual symbol.

- **Guided Visualization** Meditation: This meditation practice is another popular form of meditation and requires the meditator to follow the guidance of a speaker and visualize a scene that brings them soothing energy and peace. This is most effective when it is a vivid image that involves all five senses. For example, you can depict a peaceful forest scene where you can hear the leaves dancing in the wind, see the dappled sunlight, feel the breeze, smell the fresh pine, and taste the dew on your lip.

- **Mantra** Meditation: A mantra is a repetitive phrase, affirmation, sentence, or sound that you speak to clear the mind. This can be the universal sound of peace "om", a compassionate phrase "Om mani padme hum", or a phrase that symbolizes what you'd like more of in your life... "I am safe; I am secure; I am loved."

- **Moving** Meditation: This practice is being in motion as you meditate. Sometimes it is done in silence, sometimes with a mantra, other times people bring chi into their body. The intention is to be focused whether you are on the beach, in the forest, or walking a labyrinth.

- **Loving-Kindness** Meditation: This meditative practice asks the meditator to focus on the feelings of love and acceptance and send this energy to both themselves and the universe. Its aim is to encourage a more loving awareness of self-love in the world. To act with love and kindness throughout life to make the world a better, kinder place.

- **Progressive** Meditation: This is also known as body scan meditation and holds the purpose to relieve physical and mental tension within the body. The meditator must focus on their body, scanning the sensations from the top of their head to the tips of their toes. As they progress downward, they must try to soften and relax every part of their body. Another form of this practice is to imagine a white, cleansing light moving through your body in a progressive form to release all stored tension and energy.

The best way to cultivate a meditation routine is to learn about your Ayurveda dosha and find out the times of the day your dosha responds best to exercise or relaxation. You can begin practicing meditation for 10 minutes and build up from that. In terms of anxiety, meditation is a brilliant way to calm the mind and to let go of thoughts negatively impacting you. Over time meditation can become one of the best tools you can use to gain control over your mind and thoughts. A peaceful mind can be a challenge at the beginning, once achieved, you can use this tool to overcome your anxiety.

YOGA HELPS ANXIETY

Yoga started about 5,000 years ago in India, as the movement portion of Ayurveda. It is intended to unite the body, mind, and spirit. It's used to promote healthy functioning of organs, improve flexibility and muscle resilience, gain strength, and increase balance. However, it is also used as a form of movement that connects the breath and body to the mind, helping relieve anxiety, muscle tension, and often makes it easier to sleep.

Yoga postures, called asanas, are used to release tension in the body and mind. It soothes the nervous system and boosts the immune system. Yoga also lengthens and stretches the muscles, helping let go of stored energy that can relate into emotional tension.

Here are a few forms of yoga. Again, not all of them originated with ayurveda, yoga has evolved and grown over thousands of years.

Vinyasa Yoga: This is a flow yoga which focuses on moving in time with the breaths inhale and exhale. It is a relatively fast-paced practice that is considered more of a power yoga than many of the other forms.

Hatha Yoga: This is a slow-paced practice that focuses on the breath and grounding postures to improve balance.

Iyengar Yoga: This type of yoga is all about alignment and realigning your body and mind. Poses are held for an extended time. Originated in the early 1900's. It is ideal for injuries.

Kundalini Yoga: This practice focuses on releasing energy. It works the core muscles and marries breath with movement, often including the chanting of mantras. Kundalini practice began in India around 500 BC.

Prenatal Yoga: This form of yoga is designed specifically for pregnant people who wish to achieve physical and mental benefits without harming their baby. This emphasis became more common in the mid 20th century.

Anusara Yoga: This style of movement focuses on each body part to create more awareness of the soul, mind, and body connection. This is a tangent of Iyengar Yoga that began in the 1980's.

According to an article in the Yoga Journal Ayurveda and Asana: Yoga Poses for Your Health. The author, Halpern states that Ayurveda and Yoga are so closely intertwined that while Ayurveda is the art of staying healthy through balance in the mind and body, yoga is the art of preparation for the body and mind to receive enlightenment. 'According to Vedic scholar David Frawley, "Yoga is the practical side of the Vedic teachings, while Ayurveda is the healing side." In practice, both paths overlap.' (Halpern, 2007) In order to find the yoga practice that is best for you it is beneficial to determine where your imbalance is originating. Once you know this you can practice the form of yoga best suited to bring you balance.

According to an article in the Yoga Journal Ayurveda and Asana: Yoga Poses for Your Health, Mark Halpern discusses his experience as a doctor practicing Ayurvedic medicine. He mentioned a patient who was still suffering from neck pain and nervousness after 6 years of yoga. She didn't understand why she was still having issues. Halpern was able to review the yoga exercises she was practicing only to discover that she was actually aggravating the energies of her body and that a slight change to the asanas she practiced provided more harmony, creating balance in her body and allowing her to eliminate the neck pain and nervousness she was experiencing (Halpern, 2007).

Breathing exercises are an integral component of Ayurveda, they are often incorporated into meditation and yoga. We will not delve into this approach to wellness, yet we strongly recommended those with anxiety discuss breathing options with an Ayurveda doctor.

DAILY PURIFICATION

Snana is the Ayurveda word for a bathing ritual that occurs either shortly before sunrise or shortly before sunset. Charaka Samhita is one of two ancient foundational texts on Ayurveda, written between 100 BCE-200 CE. It states, "Bathing is purifying, life promoting, a destroyer of fatigue, physically removes sweat and dirt, is resuscitative and a promoter of Ojas or divine energy."

Bathing daily can have tremendous soothing and calming effects on both the mind and body. The literal sensations and actions of washing can transcend the outer layer of the body and calm the nervous system, relax muscles, and help the body destress from the day. Furthermore, it allows the mind to rinse away thoughts from the day, rejuvenate for a peaceful sleep, or find energy for the day ahead.

PANCHAKARMA TREATMENTS

Anxiety and stress are often stimulated by our daily surroundings and activities. Know that this modality offers treatments performed by one practitioner or two practitioners simultaneously. Ayurveda treatments are most effective for all illness especially those experiencing mental overload, burnout, powerlessness, exhaustion, nervousness, tension, or shoulder and neck problems. The goal of these treatments are to let the body and soul come to rest.

Although there are many Panchakarma treatments we will mention four that are most beneficial for stress, poor concentration, and anxiety (Authentic Ayurvedic Treatments In Kerala, India, n.d.).

- **Thalapothichil** - A sophisticated herb paste is created that aligns with the patient's dosha. This healing is delivered through the scalp, after it is applied to the upper half of the head. The therapy commonly improves memory, stress reduction, and calms nerves.

- **Nasyam** - This Panchakarma nasal rinsing therapy uses plant-based oils and herbs. Cleaning the nose and opening airways increases blood circulation and assists with poor concentration, and headaches.

- **Sirovasthi** - Commonly referred to as "head oil bath" because warm oil with herbs is poured into a unique hat on top of the head. The herbal remedy is customized for each patient. Since the oil covers the scalp, it benefits high blood pressure, depression, migraines, and more.

- **Sirodhara** - This classic cleansing therapy has an even stream of warm herbal oil, or herbal milk, that flows from side to side over a patient's forehead. The container, swings in a gentle rhythm from the temple on one side to the other. Acknowledged to be one of the most soothing treatments. This impactful treatment benefits memory loss, headaches, stress, mental tension, physical tension, and insomnia.

SOOTHE ANXIETY WITH HERBS

Ayurveda also relies heavily on medicinal herbs. In cooperation with an Ayurvedic practitioner we encourage you to track the benefits of the herbs you use and discuss what is best. Teas can have a stronger impact than anticipated. During Ayurvedic treatments herbs are combined in pindas or are added to water, oil, or milk to seep through the skin and provide additional medicinal effects. The uses of herbs follow the belief that certain plants hold properties that can both help release stress, irritability, muscle tension, and enhance concentration when you restore balance. This approach has been utilized for thousands of years and is still available in the today.

Anxiety calming herbs include (Budd, 2019):

- Holy Basil: This is, as its namesake suggests, considered to be one of the most divine and sacred plants in India. It's used to protect the patient against anxiety and emotional stress. It can be consumed in a tea form, applied as a gel, or taken in a powder form. It soothes the nervous system and is considered to be one of the best herbs as an antianxiety, antioxidant, and anti-stress medicine.

- Ashwagandha: This warming herb promotes emotional balance and grounding. Physically, it bolsters thyroid activity, which has a large impact on emotions and has shown effectiveness for insomnia and anxiety. However, it is not to be used regularly.

- Gotu Kola: This plant has been utilized both in ancient Chinese and Indian medicine and holistic healing practices. It's incredibly effective when it comes to focus, memory, nerve damage, and can further impact anxiety and stress levels.

- Bacopa: This is widely used to calm the restless mind and has recently been proven to assist those with attention deficit hyperactivity disorder (ADHD). It also bolsters cognitive abilities and helps one regain control over their emotional state.

Overall, Ayurveda has been around for thousands of years and has withstood the test of time. Still widely popular, this holistic healing method from India is incredibly useful when it comes to healing anxiety and soothing stress levels. Working with a licensed practitioner to shift a few habits or dramatically changing your lifestyle integrates healthy nutrition, movement, bathing daily, herbs, and / or panchakarma treatments. Studies show this in depth, holistic approach can find the source of your concerns and provide relief. Anxiety, irritation, and concentration loss may be replaced with energy and peacefulness.

Reflection

Is all or part of Ayurveda, meditation, yoga, herbs, panchakarma treatments, or bathing daily tools you want to incorporate in your life?

- How deep is your illness? If it is deep and debilitating, are you ready to alter your lifestyle?

- If your ailments are lighter, is there a portion of Ayurveda you want to include in your life?

- Are you willing to find and meet with an Ayurveda practitioner? Where will you look for them?

- Write down ways you are willing to integrate Ayurveda, specific times, and days of the week.

- Establish your intention and how you will track the impact of your new life.

Notes & things to remember....

CHAPTER SIX

— : —

ANIMAL THERAPY CALMS ANXIETY

*With this chapter we will shift from ancient medicine to
a newer modality that became incorporated into clinical
settings in the 1960's, Animal Therapy. Be aware if you have
pet allergies this may not be an option for you. Many of us are
fortunate to be able to hug, cuddle, and love animals. This
type of interaction stimulates the senses of see, hear, touch,
and smell. You will learn how animal therapy has changed
someone's life, the research that validates this approach, and
consider ways you can get connected to other creatures.*

A Story Of Calming Connection

Juli couldn't handle it anymore; her anxiety became too much for her to
bear. However, she was terrified of leaving her house, driving, or seeing
other people. Juli's grandmother had to accompany her to a therapist
in a desperate attempt to seek out help. All in all, Juli's anxiety had
gained control over her every move, and she was left caged in her body
as a result. Juli was assessed and prescribed medication, and then sent to
attend a cognitive behavioral therapy course to understand her mindset

(Schwartz, n.d.). She made notes of her thoughts, triggers, and emotions as she went through her days and was able to observe how her own thinking led her down the road where the destination was full-blown anxiety or a panic attack. She adopted mindfulness practices such as breathwork and meditation to calm her mind, and she began the road to improvement. Every day was a step in the right direction: Though it was a slow step, she was moving. However, she found bumps along the way and often found herself resorting back to old unhealthy habits (Schwartz, n.d.).

Then Juli was introduced to Mingo, a fully trained psychiatric golden retriever. From the very second Juli set eyes on Mingo, her shoulders relaxed, her face softened, Juli felt calm and at ease. At first touch, the two found an instant bond. Mingo gently nudged Juli, and Juli gave Mingo a big squeeze. Every therapy session after their first encounter, Mingo was present for Juli. The dog sat next to Juli, head gently leaning on her legs, while Juli softly stroked Mingo's fur coat. "There is something so reassuring about having a dog in your lap when you panic. It's like all your anxiety melts right off and onto them," says Juli. However, when Juli left Mingo, she felt a wave of anxiety return in ebbs and flows. So, her therapist eventually found her the perfect companion: Lily. Lily was an adopted puppy who Juli trained to be a service dog. It wasn't easy, and it took some time to get where they needed to be, but finally, Lily and Juli were trained, partnered, and life companions (Schwartz, n.d.).

Juli's life completely changed. She felt safe when Lily was with her life, and she had constant emotional support. Juli often left her home to explore the world with Lily and even started working again as she mustered the strength to overcome her internal battles, with Lily by her side. Today, Juli and Lily travel around as emblems of hope for those suffering with severe and acute anxiety (Schwartz, n.d.).

Animal Therapy Overview

Animals and humans have been intricately and innately intertwined for thousands of years. In nearly every human civilization, pets have been involved. From the cats of ancient Egypt to horses in ancient Rome, over the years of evolution, we have been able to cultivate a strong and powerful symbiotic relationship with animals.

It is uncertain which were the first domesticated animals, as it's challenging to track what was happening 10,000 years ago. If we accept that animals were tamed thousands of years prior for meat, milk, and hides - Mesopotamia has some of the earliest indicators that goats, sheep, chicken were domesticated. Horses and oxen were most likely domesticated early on, as they were utilized for transportation and strength. It's believed that dogs and humans found mutual acceptance as they could help each other hunt, eat, and survive.

Over the years, as the bond between humans and animals grew, pets became a norm in society and their evolution has joined that of humans to create one of the most powerful interspecies relationships of all time.

For countless years animals have been part of emotional healing methods. Animals were first recommended as therapy pets for those suffering from mental illness. Patients were able to connect with the animals and learn self-control, responsibility, and empathy when looking after one. For physical illnesses and diseases, therapy animals were seen to have increasingly positive effects on the healing process of those suffering. In the 1970's the first research efforts on the effects of animal therapy and emotional support were conducted. The blood pressure of a patient was assessed both before and after the introduction of pets, and every single time pets were introduced, the patient's blood pressure lowered significantly.

Today, animals are woven into the tapestry of human existence. They are the threads that create a sense of comfort and security, while satisfying universal desires of companionship and love. Dogs and cats are the most popular household pets. However, due to this unwavering bond between humans and animals, many different types of animals have become instrumental in fighting anxiety, stress, and depression.

The Benefits of Animal Therapy

The objective of animal therapy is to strengthen human physical, emotional, cognitive, and social functioning to achieve a higher level of performance. Animal therapy also offers a connection or bond with an animal, even if it's just petting for a time, promoting even more significant benefits.

Petting an animal improves immune systems and functioning. The enhanced positive psychological effects from close encounters with therapy animals has been studied, confirming effects on how our bodies respond to external diseases and infections. In some cases, it vastly improves the immune system and therefore makes us stronger to fight off foreign invaders. Furthermore, it has been proven that creating a physical or emotional connection with an animal, such as a dog or cat, lowers blood pressure. It instantly, and over time, combats emotions, feelings, and sensations of overwhelm, either from anxiety or depression. Even if there is no physical touch, animals can lower blood pressure and invite a sense of calm within people. This can be achieved by watching animal videos as well as thinking about animals. The interaction between animals and humans evaporates fierce feelings of loneliness, diminishing this cause of anxiety and depression. We all need to feel loved and accepted in this world an animal can fulfill both of these needs. It has been proven that even receiving a weekly visit from an animal can combat feelings of loneliness (Johnson, 2020).

Dolphins have proven that animal intervention can be even more effective and efficient than pharmaceutical medication for those suffering from depression. In children, especially those who battle social anxiety, pets have been known to dramatically decrease the release of cortisol, while improving morale, spirit, and energy levels. Furthermore, in journal entries of adolescent patients fighting anxiety, the patients reported to have feelings of happiness and feeling uplifted when a therapy pet is involved. They are more likely and able to share their problems and thoughts, while feeling calm as though they have a best friend to confide in (Johnson, 2020).

On a physical health level, therapy animals can improve cardiovascular health. Animal therapy also decreases the need for medication in some instances and regulates breathing for those who are feeling overwhelmed. In fact, petting an animal is known to release phenylethylamine, the hormone that is released when we eat and enjoy chocolate. In addition, this animal connection also releases serotonin, the ultimate mood-enhancing hormone. Animals help people of all ages and backgrounds relax, decreasing muscle tension and calm a racing mind. Not only do the physical interactions with animals have physical benefits but also encourage physical activity and promote a healthier lifestyle (Johnson, 2020). Animals need exercise, especially dogs, and owners are required to go out, to walk their dog, buy their food, and socialize. These basic needs are often not being met in individuals suffering from anxiety and depression, Research has found that dog owners often place the well-being of their pet over their own health. This compassionate companion helps people to learn what they actually need to do for their highest good.

In terms of mental health, animals provide comfort, satisfy the need for connection and acceptance, and decrease feelings of loneliness and misunderstanding. They further provide an increased mental stimulation, often helping those suffering from head or brain injuries and diseases such as Alzheimer's. The presence of an animal, especially one with a calm and soothing yet happy temperament, is an ideal way to "break the ice" between patient and therapist. Animal Therapy essentially bridges the gap and allows for each session and the overall therapeutic experience to be the best it can be, helping the therapist make more accurate decisions on how to treat the patient. The unwavering, nonjudgmental love, attention, and affection animals provide the patient offer the means to practice proper social and communicative skills, further aiding them in the real world (Johnson, 2020).

Therapy Animals And Their Training

Animal therapy is widely utilized around the world for various diseases, illnesses, and emotional support. It harnesses the power of the bonds created between humans and animals, usually through domesticated pets such as cats, dogs, rabbits, birds, and horses. The animals chosen for therapy training are chosen based on their temperament and often undergo the necessary training to become certified therapy animals.

It's important to note the difference between the type of support animals available and how they are taught to assist humans. A service animal, usually a dog, is trained to provide particular skills that help a person with disabilities on a daily basis. For example, someone who is blind or paraplegic has a dog that sees and notifies them of danger or picks things up for them. Whereas someone who has diabetes would utilize a service dog to alert them when they require medicine (Everything About Emotional Support Animals, n.d.).

Psychiatric service dogs (PSD) are also specially trained and assist people with mental illness or a learning disability that includes PTSD, anxiety, and depression. With the cooperation of the PSD, and the dog's ability to perform specific tasks, offers an individual with disabilities the ability to live a more independent life. The webmd.com site provides examples of how a trained PSD can be advantageous to someone with anxiety:

- Anticipate signs and symptoms of anxiety attacks before they start

- Distract you during an anxiety attack so that you can calm down

- Apply physical pressure with its body to help calm you down

- Warn others to give you space

- Get your medication during an anxiety attack

- Give you a sense of safety with their presence

- Alert others for help if they sense that you're in danger (What Are Psychiatric Service Dogs?, 2020)

Emotional support animals (ESA) do not need any special training and can be any pet that is a domesticated animal such as a cat, dog, bird, or rabbit, who provides comfort. If a therapist, psychologist, or psychiatrist prescribes the presence of an animal for the mental health of a patient, their pet can become an ESA. This often occurs to decrease a person's anxiety.

Now that we've seen a few examples of how animals help patients of all kinds either cope with or alleviate ailments, of a physical or mental nature, we can seriously consider incorporating animals into our own lives. There is a wide range of animal species used in animal therapy, which includes dogs, cats, horses, rabbits, guinea pigs, dolphins, hamsters, and reptiles. Animal therapy is used in myriad types of environments.

The process often includes the animal handler, who has trained and looked after the therapy animal. The handlers work under the guidance of doctors and therapists to ensure that the goals of each session are met. There are various groups and organizations who take care of either the training and pet care or who act as a bridge between patient and therapy animal. The therapy animal has to undergo evaluation to make sure they are suitable and within the correct temperament to provide support to those in need and continue to be healthy during the therapy process.

Some of these groups and organizations are:

- Pet Partners (Pet Partners, 2021)

- Wide Open Pets (Wide Open Pets, 2021)

- American Veterinary Medical Association (Service, emotional support, and therapy animals, n.d.)

Animals and humans have shared a cherished bond and connection for many years. They have evolved seemingly together and stood strong through all the tests of time. Today animals are widely perceived to be essential to human life and existence. After all, as the saying goes, "dog is a man's best friend", and it's scientifically proven to ring true. More than science, this unwavering and heart centered bond between humans and animals makes life more meaningful. The next time you are feeling down, overwhelmed, anxious, or just need a pick-me-up, a cuddly animal could be just the thing that turns you around and provides some playful time.

Reflection

Is Animal Therapy for your? Acknowledge if you have allergies to any animals try other modalities. If connection calms your nerves, consider four legged animals to fulfill that need.

- Is animal therapy a modality you would like to use to control your anxiety?

- Are you willing to consider your interaction with animals as therapy?

- Do you have a connection to animals? What type of animal?

- Do you have your own pets? If so, can you reserve more structured time with them?

- What days of the week and time of day will you reserve for your healing with animals?

- If you do not have your own pet, can you walk a neighbor's dog or care for their cat while they are at work? Are you willing to volunteer at the local animal shelter?

- How do you see animal interaction bettering your life?

- How will you measure if it is helping you?

Notes & things to remember....

CHAPTER SEVEN

—•—

ENERGY SESSIONS SHIFT ANXIETY

Your body knows how to take care of itself better than anyone else, for this reason Energy Therapy is a viable, alternative healing option. This modality interacts with the body, mind, heart, and spirit during a session. When you are with a practitioner or practicing self-care exercises, Energy Therapy opens energy flow through your chakras to promote balance and well-being. We will introduce you to valuable research related to military with PTSD, do our best to describe how energy therapy flows through chakras and meridians, as well as give you an idea as to how a session transpires.

Energy Therapy and PTSD Research

Post-traumatic stress disorder (PTSD) has become a prevalent concern for many with anxiety. PTSD is also a common and persistent problem especially in military populations. Many soldiers who do not meet clinical cutoffs for PTSD immediately upon return from deployment, have symptoms escalate to clinical levels up to 12 months post deployment. Over time, substance use disorders, depression, and interpersonal conflicts increase substantially for these soldiers, plus physical health related consequences such as, increased risk for hypertension and diabetes often flare up. Although soldiers are more likely to report mental health issues, they are significantly less likely to engage in mental health services.

A randomized controlled study was done at the Marine Corps Base Camp in Camp Pendleton, California with soldiers experiencing one or more PTSD Symptoms. The trial compared soldiers with PTSD receiving Healing Touch (HT) and guided imagery (GI) treatments versus the usual treatment of psychotherapy (including cognitive behavior therapy, biofeedback, and relaxation training) and often medications. The HT and GI group received 6 treatments of 1 hour each, over a 3-week period in addition to standard care. The three specific HT techniques utilized were Chakra Connection intended to simulate movement of vital energy through the body, Mind Clearing to stimulate mental relaxation, and Chakra Spread to promote deep healing for emotional and physical pain. GI is a complementary therapy that utilizes visualization to induce a state of deep relaxation, the GI recording used was Healing Trauma (PTSD) – Healthy Journeys by Belleruth Naparstek. This recording utilizes affirmations and imagery to enhance relaxation, reduce negative emotions attributed to PTSD (such as terror and shame), and promote self-esteem and a sense of protection. Although participants were given the GI recording and encouraged to listen to it at least once a day. No one followed up on use, meaning the incorporation of this GI outside the HT session was not tracked.

PTSD symptoms markedly declined for the HT group. A decrease in depression was noted over time. Mental health quality of life indicators increased over time. "Results indicate significant and substantial reductions in PTSD symptoms, depression and cynicism as well as improved mental quality of life for those receiving the intervention", Healing Touch, and Meditation. "Beck Depression Inventory (BDI) has been found to be optimal in predicting major depressive disorder (18); thus, the pre-post drop from 26.1 to 16.4 for the intervention group also suggests a clinically meaningful reduction in depression." "The decrease in cynicism, for participants receiving the intervention, is particularly noteworthy. Reports of higher cynicism are common among active-duty combat soldiers and likely related to issues of perceived stigma and negative beliefs about traditional mental health care that appears to hinder these soldiers from seeking help from mental health sources for PTSD." This indicates the possibility of implementing such interventions in military health settings to help quickly reduce the suffering of returning active-duty military suffering from combat-related PTSD and depression (Shamini, et al., 2012).

Energy Therapy Overview

The value of Energy Therapy is its association with the energy that surrounds us, everything in the universe is made up of energy. The different vibrations, speeds, and frequencies of energy make up matter. In the world, different vibrations affect matter in various ways, such as the gravitational pull of the moon and how those vibrations affect the tides of the ocean. Within our bodies, our heartbeats are the pulse of life itself, and breathing rates are constant evidence to the rhythmic vibrations we create without a thought. If you walk into a room and are greeted with a smile, light energy, and a calm demeanor you have experienced a positive energy exchange. When you are in a room and someone walks in and you feel they are dark, heavy, negative you may choose to walk in a different direction, you experienced a uncomfortable negative energy exchange. Energy is not visible, yet we generate and receive it continually.

Healing Touch (HT), Therapeutic Touch, and Reiki are the most common energy modalities available today. The flow of energy through your body when compromised, can cause uncomfortable feelings and painful affects to your physical and emotional state. The goal of Energy Therapy is to open energy blocked in your chakras or meridians and invite the energy to return to its natural flow, from which it can attend to healing your body itself.

"Healing Touch is a relaxing, nurturing, heart-centered energy therapy that uses gentle, intentional touch that assists in balancing physical, emotional, mental, and spiritual well-being." (Healing Beyond Borders, n.d.) In the 1980's the founder Janet Mentgen, RN, BSN compiled a series of standardized, noninvasive techniques that help to clear, energize, and balance the human and environmental energy fields. Classes began being taught in 1989 so Healing Touch practitioners could assist clients in practicing a coherent and balanced energy field, supporting their inherent ability to heal. Healing Touch is safe for everyone of all ages and may be integrated with standard medical care (Healing Beyond Borders, n.d.). Because HT was founded by a nurse, the training is more consistent than Reiki. Healing Touch (HT) is classified by the National Institute of Health as a biofield therapy and nursing intervention.

Therapeutic Touch is intended to help individuals relax, relieve their pain and heal more quickly. According to The University of Michigan, "Therapeutic touch is thought to promote healing through restoring harmony to a person's energy fields (Staff, 2020)." Utilizing a calm mind, the practitioner places their hands either above or lightly touching the patient's body working to bring their energy fields into balance.

Reiki originated in Japan in the early stages of 1920 with Mikao Usui's teachings. Having been brought up with Buddhism, Shintoism, and Taoism, Usui had many spiritual influences and knowledge that helped shape his beliefs. Marrying these together gave birth to what we know to be Reiki (Rand, 2000). The words are derived from the Japanese words rei, meaning universal or something that is everywhere, and ki, which translates to life energy. Usui taught the art to only 16 students in his lifetime, one of his graduates, Chujiru Hayashi, was given Usui's blessing to open his very own Reiki center in Tokyo. Madame Takata became his student, and she was the one who brought this method of energy healing to Europe and America (Rand, 2000).

Today, across the globe there are up to one million Reiki practitioners (Rand, n.d.) and over 90,000 people who have taken level one or more of Healing Touch. Thousands of success stories and research tout the effectiveness of energy healing. First and foremost, energy work advances harmony and balance within the body, mind, spiritual and emotional levels. While this works to release and relax the muscles, it also unblocks stored energy, helping enhance memory, and eases both physical and mental pain. The energy practice is effective when it comes to clearing the mind, soothing sensations of anxiety, and stress which also promotes healthier sleeping habits. Finally, the ultimate purpose and design of this holistic healing is focused on releasing what is in the way of your body's energy system to return to a healthier state and improve self-healing.

Understanding Personal Energy

Ancient philosophies were the first to describe energy over 4000 years ago. Although energy is hard to explain with words, let's set a context as to how different beliefs conceptualize this word. Ayurveda shares an ancient Sanskrit word for vital life force, Prana. The ancient Indian culture addresses the human system as based on the properties of "Chakras", the wheels of energy. While Chi (Qi or Ki) refers to the energy of life itself or life force energy in Traditional Chinese Medicine (TCM) and Japanese Energy Healing. TCM considers "Meridians" as the pathways of energy within the body that carry Qi, the life force energy for wellbeing. The western culture considers the Biofield or Aura as descriptors of the human energy system that integrates both the physical body and energetic fields surrounding the body. Now we will delve into the details of each of these concepts that integrate energy and health.

Chakras are included in the training for all the Energy Therapists we are discussing. Chakras provide an ancient approach to start exploring energy. There are different philosophies as to how many chakras there are, however, everyone agrees on the seven major chakra points in the body: the crown, third eye, throat, heart, solar plexus, sacral, and root. The concept of chakras was developed in ancient India, dating back to as long as 15,000 BC. It follows the energy flow of the body. These points are believed to emulate wheels turning that move cyclically to link our bodies, with our organs, the endocrine glands and nervous system, all of which connect with our emotions. In a more scientific study of chakras, these points are in fact where some of the major bundles of human nerves sit (Majumdar, 2018) (Shah, 2020). This is a portion of information about each chakra, further research can open a wealth of knowledge.

- The **root chakra** is located below the base of your spine and signifies grounded energy, stability, and survival. Color is red. Potential Dysfunction: If this chakra is blocked, possible problems include constipation, eating disorder, lack of energy, confusion, depression, immune related disorder, hypertension, chronic lower back pain. Positive Function: Security, Safety, Vitality.

- The **sacral chakra** that is located above the pubic bone and below the navel, provides energy for pleasure, sexuality, and creativity. Color is orange. Potential Dysfunction: A blocked sacral chakra can cause lower back pain, sciatica, urinary tract infections, impotence, dysfunction of reproductive organs, loss of appetite, resentment, codependency, poor relationship skills. Positive Function: Trust in one's self, positive self-image, able to establish close bonds in relationship.

- The **solar plexus chakra** is below the diaphragm, above the umbilicus it energizes personal power, self-esteem, and confidence. Color is yellow. Potential Dysfunction: Blockages to this chakra can cause stomach ulcers, eating problems and digestive disorders. Other potential deficiencies may include diabetes, pancreatitis, arthritis and allergies. Positive Function: Personal power, Self-esteem, sense of direction, good digestion, self-talk is positive, will-power, assertiveness.

- The **heart chakra** is located at the mid-chest aligned with the heart, it symbolizes love, connection, and compassion. Color is green. Potential Dysfunction: A blocked heart chakra can mean heart or lung problems, asthma, allergies, immune deficiency, dysfunctional relationships, high or ;ow blood pressure, tension between shoulder blades. Positive Function:

Transformation through unconditional love, forgives easily, harmony, compassion, able to give and receive unconditional love.

- The **throat chakra** is located in the notch at the base of the throat, it represents communication our ability to speak our highest truth. Color is light blue. Potential Dysfunction: a blocked throat chakra can display problems vocalizing, throat problems, mouth ulcers, laryngitis, ear infections, headaches, thyroid problems, hoarseness, bronchitis, unexpressive, holding back creative ideas. Positive Function: Clear communication, creativity, expressive verbally.

- The **third eye chakra** is located between the eyebrows, it is the center of our intuition. Color is indigo blue. Potential Dysfunction: a blockage can cause sinus and headaches problems, brain tumors, stroke, learning disabilities, lack of concentration, hearing issues, spinal disorders, difficulty with details, poor insight, critical and judgmental, eyestrain. Positive Function: Intuitive skills, insight, wisdom, compassion, sense of humor.

- The **crown chakra** on the top center area of the head, provides our point of enlightenment and spiritual connection. Color is Violet. Potential Dysfunction: a blockage in this area can generate frustration, migraine headaches, inability to learn, destructive feelings, depression, confusion, feeling lost, disconnected. Positive Function: Alignment with Higher will, Universal consciousness, body system in harmony, higher sense perception, connection to our high selves, others, and ultimately to the divine.

(sources: Nanda, n.d.; www.thehindu.com; and Healing Beyond Borders EducationCommittee, 2010).

Most Energy Therapists are mindful of meridians in addition to chakras. There is respect for the beliefs of Traditional Chinese Medicine (TCM), the value of energetic systems throughout our bodies, a healing philosophy based on harmony, and the interrelatedness of organs and meridians within our body. Understanding acupuncture meridians can be extremely useful, we encourage you to do more research if you are interested. We will be doing a very high-level introduction, so you have a simple understanding of how working with meridians to enhance your energy flows can help address anxiety, irritability, lack of sleep, and more.

TCM meridians are channels that your qi or energy flows through. They are networks throughout the body comparable to the circulatory system from western medicine however meridians are not physical (Acupuncture & Massage College, 2017). There are 12 major meridians that span the body:

- Lung Meridian- Regulates the respiratory system including qi. It manages the gas and water within the body and externally. Imbalance presents as shortness of breath, cough, allergies, grief, or depression.

- Large Intestine Meridian- Regulates how your body absorbs water, digestion, and the extraction of waste. Circulation in the lungs support bowel movements. Imbalance presents constipation or shortness of breath.

- Stomach Meridian- Receives food then breaks it down and digests it. Then it proceeds to the spleen so nutrients can assimilate in the blood. Together the digestive process is complete. Imbalance presents as nausea, stomach ache, mental illness.

- Spleen (Pancreas) Meridian- Manages the process of converting food nutrients into the blood. As it transports nutrients through the blood it removes impurities. Cleansing the blood is an important role for one's immune system and also helps muscles function with elasticity and strength. Imbalance appears with unexpected bleeding or tiredness or weakness.

- Heart Meridian- Responsible for blood vessels and transportation of blood within the body, as well as sweating. Also manages some mental and psychological functions. Imbalance presents with restlessness, heart palpitations, lack of or excess of sweating.

- Small Intestine Meridian- Processes and allocates substances from the stomach. The nourishing portion is absorbed and passed to the spleen. Any turbid substance goes to the large intestine. Remaining watery juice goes to the badder. Paired with the Heart the small intestine dances sharing TCM fire. Imbalance presents as infrequent urination, excitability, or cold sores.

- Bladder Meridian- Releases toxins from the body. Imbalance presents as problems with bladder control.

- Kidney Meridian- Manages production of bone marrow, brain, and spinal cord while being a source of conception and growth. Imbalance presents lack of will power, impairs short term memory. Also, when there is a lack of qi in the kidneys, the bladder control is disrupted which influences incontinence.

- Pericardium Meridian- Regulates energy surrounding and protecting the heart and circulation of blood. When combined with the heart together they impact the central nervous system. Imbalance presents as unbalanced emotions and reduces mental state.

- Triple Heater (San Jiao) Meridian- Regulates the operation of all internal organs.

- Gallbladder Meridian- Accumulates bile, secondarily it transfers secretion to the digestive tract. Imbalance presents mental illness or psychosomatic disorders.

- Liver Meridian- Regulates and filters blood. Substances are moved within and excreted from of the body. Energy for managing ligaments and tendons. Imbalance presents headaches, anger, depression. (sources: The 12 Major Meridians, 2020. Twelve Main Meridians in traditional Chinese medicine, 2014. Wong, C., 2021 February 26. How Emotions and Organs Are Connected in Traditional Chinese Medicine.)

A study was done on the impact of acupuncture on the 12 meridian points versus a medication treatment for the reduction of anxiety. After 4-6 weeks it was found that a superior and faster impact was made to anxiety disorder with the use of the 12 meridian acupoints than was found in patients using clonazepam as a medication to reduce anxiety. While used in acupuncture the meridians can also be used in many forms of energy healing to alleviate anxiety (Jiu, Zhou, Li, Zhu, & Chen, 2013).

Biofields or auras have been identified as the energy that surrounds the body. The International Chiropractic Pediatric Association stated, "The biofield is composed of both measurable electromagnetic energy and hypothetical subtle energy, or chi. This structure is also referred to as the "human energy field" or "aura"...Subtle energy is to electromagnetism as water vapor is to water. Just as we do not measure water vapor with the tools we use to measure water, we can't measure subtle energy with the same tools we'd use to measure electricity. Subtle energy is higher, finer, and more diffuse; it follows slightly different laws (McKusick, 2020)."

In Biofield tuning research they found that our life experiences are stored magnetically and the biofield records and stores the emotions from those experiences. Negative emotions such as guilt, grief, anger, and anxiety can be carried around with us. Through understanding biofields we can use the ability to tap into the stressors in our biofield/aura relieving those negative emotions to find balance and remove or reduce anxiety (McKusick, 2020).

Incorporating Energy Healing

We recommend starting with a session from a certified Healing Touch or Reiki practitioner. This is a useful place to begin and send you in the best direction given the issues you are managing. Anxiety, irritability, lack of sleep, all influence the self-care recommendations given to you, to do at home.

Here is an overview of how an Energy Therapy session often unfolds. The practitioner will spend the first few minutes of the session asking what your concerns are, listening to your approach of caring for yourself, and what you want support with. An intention is set for the session. You will be asked to lie on the massage table, fully clothed, glasses and shoes removed. There is often an additional assessment with a pendulum or energetic scan so the practitioner becomes acquainted with your energy. According to the aspects you previously spoke about with the practitioner, they will place their hands either above or gently on your body. Before or during the session you can request the practitioner not touch you if it is uncomfortable. Often clients feel a sense of deep relaxation. You might be feeling a feather of warmth gliding over you, or your fingers and limbs may experience a tingling sensation. This is your body shifting into rest and rejuvenation, where it has the ability to heal. This is when the body begins healing itself, which helps boost the immune system, balance mental and emotional states, to assist in the body's detoxification process.

Depending on your current state practitioners may offer energy so you feel more grounded, fulfilled, and energized. Alternatively, they may assist your energy in moving out to release the highest amount of overwhelm, uncontrollable sensations, or tension. This shift of energy impacts your body, mind, heart, and spirit because most of our emotions and feelings are physically stored in parts of our body. When we release emotional energy there is a calmer connection within one's body, often a huge sigh of relief is felt in one's mind as well. The session ends with a discussion about your experience so you both gain a better understanding of what sensations you felt and what was most beneficial. Your practitioner will discuss self-care exercises and next steps personalized for you. After a session it is recommended that you drink water, remain highly attuned to your body, and the shift of your mental state. The aftereffects for many people are to enjoy more productivity, a calmer mind, and a better night of sleep.

Energy Therapy is also used in clinics as an additional means of pain management and anti-stress therapy. In 2010, a research study was hosted by Yale University students and their report was published in the Journal of the American College of Cardiology. The researchers found that just a mere 20 minutes of Reiki dramatically increased the mood and mental state of recent heart attack patients. It also significantly lowered their heart rates and helped them manage both the emotional and physical pain (Friedman et al., 2010).

A study was done for nursing students in their junior year at Widener University in Chester, Pennsylvania. 37 students were given the State Trait Anxiety Inventory (STAI) assessment. After completing the initial assessment, they were given a 50-minute healing touch session and provided with a second STAI assessment to complete. This study found a decrease in anxiety when this was done. (Klein, Krouse, & Lowe, 2014).

Specifically related to anxiety, Energy Therapy can help in many different ways. First, it invites patients to be fully present in their body, with this heightened sense of awareness, patients are more likely to identify what is triggering them. As a holistic tool Energy Therapy patients often notice their ability to be calm and quiet minded after a session.

Reflection

Consider incorporating the benefits of energy therapy.

- Is Energy Therapy a modality you would like in your toolbox to manage your anxiety?

- How will you find Healing Touch and Reiki practitioners in your area?

- What days of the week and time of day will you reserve for sessions with a practitioner or energy focused self-care?

- How will you measure if energy therapy is helping you?

Notes & things to remember....

Chapter Eight

— · —

Sound Healing Releases Anxiety

Our sense of hearing influences our actions constantly, this chapter uncovers the value of sound as a healing therapy. Some people with anxiety prefer not to touch or be touched as it creates overstimulation. The power of vibrations from sound can be a viable alternative to release unwanted sensations. Read further to hear how a woman overcame her anxiety with Tibetan bowls. Learn how early sound was an integral part of society, when it became a healing mechanism, and ways you can incorporate sound vibration for a healthier life.

A Story About Sound Healing

Danielle Bauman was riddled with anxiety. Whenever she started to feel a panic attack creeping its way in and taking control, she would play music to herself either to soothe or to encourage tears to release some of her worked-up energy, but it wasn't enough. She hated her job and wasn't enjoying the direction her life was going. In a desperate attempt to calm herself down, Bauman attended a restorative yoga session. While the slow movement and breathing helped ease her rushing mind, it was the introduction of the Tibetan sound bowls that truly changed something inside of her. "Literally the first time I heard these bowls, I sat up, and I cried," she said. ". . . I didn't even know what was happening to me, but I could feel something in my body for the first time in a long time (Petitt, 2020)." The power of her very first sound healing and sound therapy session impacted Bauman so much so that she immediately started her certification for sound healing. Today, Bauman is a sound healing practitioner and therapist, healing people through vibrations (Petitt, 2020).

Sound Healing Overview

Music has been utilized in numerous civilizations around the globe, mainly for healing purposes. Drumming, flutes from reeds, rattles, symbols, harps, stomping, clapping, and chanting were and still are used to create deeper connections with oneself and the world, as well as heal diseases, infections, and tension. Australian aboriginal tribesmen used their indigenous instrument, the didgeridoo, as a tool for healing over 40,000 years ago. In Tibet, ancient singing bowls were, and still are, used in Buddhist rituals, for meditation purposes, as well as healing the connection to the divine energy through the mind, body, and soul.

Sound healing is an ancient meditative practice the first written in Vedic texts, 4000 years old, where Lord Vishnu described the hum known as Aum. Then consider the harmonic frequencies you can experience when you visit ancient Egyptian pyramids, Greek Asclepian temples, Central and South American Mayan temples, Gothic cathedrals, or hear an Aboriginal didgeridoo being played. Architecture was redesigned and sculpted to capture and compose light and sound waves. Millions of people around the world, historically and today, flock to buildings with these attentive designs for guidance, spirituality, and healing.

Pythagoras, born around 569 BC in Greece, taught students how his knowledge of mathematics and music intervals could create healing sounds and harmonies, he laid out harmonic ratios. The sound harnesses the power and vibrations of assorted instruments that create a variety of healing frequencies that, in turn, heal the body and mind. Pythagoras taught his students about sound, sound waves, and how these frequencies could soothe their anger and bring them happiness.

The human body and mind parallel the teachings of Pythagoras. Since we are all made up of energy and atoms, we create our own frequencies, we can easily be moved or influenced by sound frequencies. "Each celestial body, in fact each and every atom, produces a particular sound on account of its movement, its rhythm, or vibration. All these sounds and vibrations form a universal harmony in which each element, while having its own function and character, contributes to the whole (QuoteFancy, n.d.)."

Ancient healing techniques were transferred through verbal stories, however, in 1869 music as a form of healing was actually chronicled. Many physicians in America began discovering that specific types of music aided patients with healthier blood flow and therefore promoted cell repair, stimulated brain functioning, and altered the rhythm of heart rates. Advances in sound healing continued in the times of World War II where it was harnessed and used in rehabilitation treatment for soldiers battling from post-traumatic stress disorder (PTSD). Then, in the 1950s and 60s, European doctors began noticing the profound benefits of sound as well. Sir Peter Guy Manners, a British osteopath, created a sound machine which he used to treat patients. This machine sent out vibrations and frequencies that matched the frequencies of the cells found in healthy bodies. By using this machine, unhealthy cells are influenced and started to shift into healthier ones, slowly healing the body from within (Sound Therapy, n.d.).

Today, many instruments, including the Tibetan singing bowl and didgeridoo, are still used to heal both physical and emotional ailments. Acceptance of healing from vibration is growing as its effectiveness is proven time and time again. Some people who suffer from anxiety, stress, or depression often don't like or want to be touched. Sound healing therefore offers a noninvasive approach in an extremely soothing therapy session, without speech or social interactions needed. The power of vibrations and frequencies through sound can prove to be a viable alternative that is a natural and powerful way to release anxiety.

The Science Of Sound

Sound makes up one of the most significant parts of our human experience. It fills in the gaps and adds an entirely new dimension to our environment. It is often the very first sense that is activated when you wake up and an the last before going to sleep. What is sound? How does it work? Sound is, like everything else, energy. The movement of the energy creates vibrations that then hit surfaces, causing the surrounding air to vibrate on the same frequency. This includes the air in your ears, as that air vibrates, you hear sounds.

There are two processes when it comes to sound: the physical and the psychological. The physical is what was just described, while the psychological is what and how your brain perceives each sound. For example, speech is just noise, but our brains make these sounds become language from which we gather meaning. Sound travels in waves, and different wavelengths and movements from varying instruments that produce their own set of unique waves. Combined with vibrations and frequencies, from singing to yelling, these waves of sound can have an impact on our physical and mental state.

The vibrations emitted from a sound hit our eardrums. These energies are then moved through a tunnel within the ear that is filled with fluid and hair cells. The vibrations cause the movement of these fluids, creating their very own waves and then moving the hair cells. The ear sends these auditory messages to the brain, which then gets to work on decoding the message. If there are two different noises or sounds, (i.e., music and a siren) each equipped with their own set of vibrations, the ears will take in both vibrations and the brain will find the average of these. This is one of the most common methods of sound therapy and healing. Sound healing utilizes an alpha-theta-gamma-delta range, which is a lower vibrational frequency (Vidraschu, 2018). When we are awake and highly attentive and alert, we most likely process vibrations and sound frequencies at 14–40 hertz, whereas when we are in a sleeping state, which is the best state for healing and repair, we process these sounds at only around eight hertz (Vidraschu, 2018).

This means that lower vibrations are more effective when it comes to overall healing. A lower vibrational frequency stimulates and promotes the production of serotonin. Research shows that particular sound and vibrational healing supports memory recall, halts the production of cortisol, and helps to balance one's emotional state. It also stimulates the creative state and lights up the regions of the brain responsible for imagination and creativity. In fact, when Albert Einstein's brain was analyzed while he was solving complex mathematical equations, he was in a lower frequency state, the alpha-band state. This state of lower vibration, and the process of experiencing lower frequencies, has also been proven to release nitric oxide, which is a hormone responsible for signaling muscle soothing and tension release by dilating blood vessels and increase the flow of blood itself as well as the oxygen levels (Vidraschu, 2018).

To find out the effects of sound, a group of scientists from the U.S. National Library of Medicine National Institutes of Health conducted a thorough test. Starting with the facts that sensations of stress and anxiety arise due to an individual's perception of the environmental demands. Heightened levels of stress can be detrimental to your physical health as well as your mental health. The stress effects are felt, noticed, and regulated by the central nervous system and subcortical limbic system. Since research has been conducted around sound, it has been highly evident that music initiates a myriad of cognitive processes and has an influence over stress-releasing hormones including the part of the brain and nervous system that governs sensations of warning and danger. The research project found 60 healthy females in their 20s and exposed them to stressful triggers. Once the women were found to have a substantial amount of cortisol flowing through them, they were separated into groups and given different sounds to listen to. One group was assigned rippling water noises, another soothing music, and the final group was given silence (Thoma et al., 2013).

The results were as follows. The first group, who listened to rippling water noises, were found to have the lowest amount of cortisol, closely followed by the group who listened to relaxing music. Those who were forced to listen to silence took an increasingly longer time to recover their stability than those listening to blissful vibrations. The conclusion was that music and vibrations do have healing effects on a human's nervous system and aids in a quicker recovery process (Thoma, 2013).

Another study conducted by the National Institutes of Health in 2012 divided a group of 39 people who were currently caring for family members who suffered from dementia. They were stressed and anxious from their work, with high levels of cortisol. One group was asked to listen to soothing music for 12 minutes every day for eight weeks, while the other was asked to practice a form of yoga and meditation paired with chanting for the same amount of time. The results? While the group who listened to relaxing music experienced a decrease in their cortisol levels and therefore anxiety levels, the yoga chanting group reported a significant decrease in stress and depression. While music clearly has an effect on the cognitive process, the actual vibrations that are created, and then truly felt by humans, is where the real healing happens (Purtill, 2016).

Sound Healing Methods And Benefits

Common, simple forms of sound healing and therapy include (Santos-Longhurst, 2020):

- Listening to music

- Singing with music or a choir

- Reading or listening to Poetry

- Meditating while listening to music or Guided Meditation

- Playing an instrument especially flute or drums

- Kirtan (a call and response chant to music that originated from ancient Vedic anukirtana)

- Solfeggio Frequencies (Specific tones that emit healing frequencies)

- Binaural Beats (Particular rhythmic beats that create healing vibrations)

- Vocal toning

Consider the possibilities of vibrational therapy coming from different instruments. Here are four common instruments and two ways to use one's voice to create sound healing sessions:

- Tibetan Bowl: Also referred to as singing or standing bowls, these ancient, spiritual, and sacred bowls are available at various frequencies to address different ailments, and create a sound and vibration that synchronize with our desired healing frequencies.

- Gong Bath: This ancient healing technique, originating from Asia, it cleanses and soothes the entire physical and mental body. This deep, powerful tone vibrates the entirety of the water within the body, which acts like a bath and massage for the soul.

- Tuning Fork: These instruments can be incredibly effective to tune the body back into its soothing, harmonic form. Depending on your imbalance, a specific tuning fork is chosen to align your vibrational needs in the body or mind. These forks can also rebalance and open the chakras causing a release of tension in the muscles. It is beneficial to begin this with a certified sound healer.

- Classical Music: We all know classical music and how it positively affects people. The synchronicity of the orchestra can have healing impacts on heart rates, and blood pressure. Did you know that the classical tempo helps to increase memory retention and reduce anxiety?

- Aum Chanting: "Aum" is the universal sound of peace and harmony. The sound also holds incredible healing properties as it is chanted at a low frequency, vibrating the entire body. This chant expressed in community, in person, or virtual often generates a more powerful sensation. It is generally used to stabilize the heart rate, improve blood circulation, increase oxygen levels, release muscle tension, encourage the production of endorphins, and soothe the nervous system. Overall, it's a fantastic method that requires no tools to help ease the negative sensations of stress and anxiety.

- Humming: We can all hum, and we often do when we're feeling emotions of joy and happiness. The vibrations of humming can decrease stress levels, help create stronger and healthier sleep patterns, and produce chemicals and hormones that promote calm and happiness. It can also help strengthen your sinuses by improving the airflow through your naval cavity.

As we have learned, everything in the entire world has its own vibration and frequency. Humans are made up of mostly water, and water is an incredibly efficient conductor of sounds. That's why sound is an extremely useful tool for rebalancing our physical and emotional states and finding harmony within. Now it is time to delve a bit deeper into music as the mechanism for sound healing and therapy methods that aim to soothe the soul, calm the mind, and reduce stress overall.

Music therapy offers numerous options: Neurologic music therapy uses low vibrational frequencies to help heal physical pain, as well as balance emotional states during a recovery phase or before a major treatment. This type of sound healing has been proven to be more effective than some pharmaceutical drugs aimed to achieve the same desired response in the body and brain. The Bonny Method is a technique some counselors use. It utilizes classical music, which is paired with imagery to help strengthen the connection to consciousness, thus promoting healthy growth and transformation. This has been proven to drastically improve mental states and must be done by a trained Neurologic Music Therapist (Neurologic Music Therapy, n.d.). The Nordoff-Robbins method, uses the creation of music to help children who suffer from late developmental processes and learning difficulties (Nordoff-Robbins Center for Music Therapy, n.d.).

The brainwave entrainment method. This specific technique is called entrainment and was discovered by Christina Huygens, a Dutch scientist who also invented the pendulum clock—a clock that uses weights that swing and is used for keeping time and rhythm. During the development stages, Huygens discovered that two swinging clocks, no matter how different each of the clock's rhythms might be, will eventually synchronize and match up (Spoor & Swift, 2000). When this level of entrainment happens, energy is moved between the two sources, and their energy entwines. For us, entrainment can happen when we are singing in a group. We feed off each other's energies to create one synchronized and harmonic sound or vibration. When a patient is feeling out of balance and able to experience someone else's healing sound vibrations, they are able to connect and match up to that vibration, thus shifting their energy, vibration, and frequency to one that harmonizes, promoting inner healing.

We just presented numerous ways to experience the benefits of the vibration of sound you can implement it into your daily life. If you want to feel the full benefits, you can join a sound healing class online or in your local area. Everyone's experience is different, hopefully, you will feel a state of deep relaxation. You may experience visualizations, see a variety of colors, feel a tingling sensation, or even go to a place where it feels like you are floating through space and time. Whatever your experience it can enrich your wellness.

Sound healing and therapy is beneficial for the body, mind, and soul. First and foremost, it penetrates our unseen physical frequencies and creates a soothing response on many levels. Even if nothing else happens, you will have calmed the mind, released muscle tension, and cleared your cluttered mindset. It also helps unblock chakras and release stored energy as vibrations activate energy blocks causing them to open. Such an experience is why some patients of sound therapy will often laugh or cry—a sign of energy release. Sound therapy may also boost your immune system and your overall health. It decreases the risks of heart disease and heart attacks, improves sleeping patterns, reenergizes, and relieves physical and emotional pain. Sound healing is an invigorating tool for easing anxiety and stress, balancing the mind and promoting overall wellness.

Reflection

Did you hear the benefits of sound healing? Take a moment to assess the value of sound healing for you.

- Is this a tool you would like to use regularly?

- Are you an auditory learner?

- Is music overwhelming or calming for you?

- Can you feel vibrations in your body when you hear different sounds?

- Is sound healing and experiencing frequency shifts appealing to you?

- Are you willing to find classes or practitioners offering sound healing close to home or online?

- How will you measure the impact to see if it is benefiting you?

Notes & things to remember....

CHAPTER NINE

— : —

HYPNOTHERAPY UNRAVELS ANXIETY

*Hypnotherapy is one of the modalities that must be
experienced with a trained professional. One of the strengths
of alternative medicine is the focus on the root cause, not
the symptoms. Hypnosis is a holistic option that gives the
patient the ability to unravel deep issues that can be the
constant restimulation of anxiety and its side effects. This
is not an alternative for anyone who has had a psychotic
episode or for anyone using drugs or alcohol on a regular
basis. Hypnotherapy is not an approach to be taken lightly,
as you will read there are many who have encountered
great benefits. We will also cover the science behind this
complementary medicine and describe how a session may
unfold.*

A Story About Hypnotherapy

Ilana Kaplan (2017) had not felt like herself in a while. Depression,
stress, and anxiety had a regular hold over her mind. She felt. completely
disconnected from herself and desperately missed the person she used

to be before anxiety had taken over her life. She was prescribed antidepressant medication, and while this helped for a while, it never solved the root cause of her problems (Kaplan, 2017). When family deaths occurred and Kaplan was laid off from her job, her PTSD hit again, her insomnia struck tenfold, and her OCD was almost uncontrollable. Longing to find a means of escape, Kaplan turned to something she never thought she would do in her life: hypnosis. Her very first hypnotherapy session started with talk therapy. Then, the hypnotherapist spoke to her through a 20-minute hypnotic experience. For the next eight months, Kaplan would participate in sessions and listen to a recording right before she went to sleep. The recordings didn't make sense to her, but she knew there were subconscious commands entombed within the scripted words of the recordings. Today, Kaplan feels like herself again. She recommends it to everyone and heralds the practice as one of the most enriching and life changing experiences she could have. Hypnotherapy essentially helped her reclaim her mind, regain control over her thoughts, and find her sovereignty (Kaplan, 2017).

Hypnotherapy Overview

Hypnotherapy and hypnosis may have a certain negative connotation and stigma attached to it. Used correctly, it can be a powerful tool to heal past trauma, ease anxiety, and mitigate the harmful effects of depression in the present. Hypnotherapy requires extreme focus to reach a heightened and deeper state of relaxation, which in turn helps the patient achieve an uplifted mental state and level of awareness. Some people even enter an altered mind state or trance. It's ultimately used to explore hidden memories of abuse and trauma, so that healthy habits can be instilled. Additionally, many find it a solution for breaking bad habits and a tool to rewire an anxious brain. Hypnotherapy in its essence a set of reminders to both your conscious and subconscious brain to decrease thoughts that produce anxiety and fear. It stimulates the brain to take a more positive approach and direction in life.

Hypnotherapy History

Hypnosis spans back to the ancient Egyptian and Greek civilizations. Hypnos is the Greek word for sleep, even though during hypnosis you are not asleep but rather in a higher state of conscious awareness. In fact, in these ancient civilizations, there were hypnosis centers where people could venture to seek help for their problems. Shamans across the globe used hypnosis and trance-like states to induce a state of healing.

Modern hypnosis was developed and sculpted by Austrian physician Franz Mesmer in the 18th century. His name is the basis for the term 'to mesmerize'. He created the concept, named animal magnetism, believing there was fluid through a person's body. He outlined how illnesses and diseases are results of blockages within the energy flow and state of the human body and cured them with magnets. One of Mesmer's students Marquis de Puysegir coined the process for leading clients into a 'somnambluism', a deep relaxing trance. Marquis de Puysegir identified three cardinal features that continue to be used as reference today: "Concentration of the senses of the operator, Acceptance of a suggestion from the therapist, Amnesia for events in a trance (Demant, n.d.)."

Later a Scottish doctor James Braid found object fixation fascinating. He was the first to swing a pocket watch in front of his patients to put them into a trance-like state (Hypnosis, 2021). In time, the idea of hypnotism grew across the world. Doctors and therapists from India to France started practicing with the theory as a means of pain relief and management. As hypnotherapy became more prevalent in the 1800s, French-born Émile Coué developed affirmations patients could repeat. He fiercely believed that no one could be healed, but rather, they could be given the tools to heal themselves. Thus, he believed hypnosis was one of the best means to help a patient help themselves (Hypnosis, 2021).

Finally, in 1930, American-born Clark Hull released and published his book *Hypnosis and Suggestibility*, which ultimately gave way to the growth the popular hypnotherapy people received. Today, hypnotherapy is used to treat illnesses and disease, to end bad habits like addiction to smoking and drinking, and to alleviate psychological trauma and feelings of stress. In therapy, hypnosis is used to encourage a shift in one's consciousness to help the patient be more open about their issues and to see it from a new perspective (Hypnosis, 2021).

The Science Of Hypnotherapy

There are two main forms of hypnotherapy: suggestion and analysis.

Suggestion therapy is utilized with a patient whose mind can easily respond to suggestions. They will heed the requests of the therapist while induced in a heightened state of consciousness or trance. This particular method is generally used to halt the continuation of bad habits, such as a smoking or drinking addiction. It also has the power to change to healthier habits, giving patients a much-needed nudge in the right direction and assisting with motivation.

Analysis therapy is specifically used to uncover and reveal issues of trauma. Many of us who have trauma tend to keep the memories and triggers of trauma locked away deep inside, never fully accepting, exposing, or dealing with the root of the problem. Hypnotherapy allows those dealing with trauma to unveil their problems in their conscious and unconscious memories. This method, also known as regression therapy, puts the patient in a trance-like altered state, and then explores and analyzes the patient's traumatic past, events, memories, and people that may still be causing them damage and harm now. The end goal is for the patient to face the trauma and move past it for optimal health and mental well-being and to release the burden and clutches of anxiety, stress, and post-traumatic stress disorder.

At Stanford University, Heidi Jiang and her colleagues (2017) conducted a research study to further deepen their understanding of hypnosis. First, they screened 545 healthy individuals to assess whether they were able to be hypnotized and if their brains responded well to suggestions. Only 57 out of the group of 545 were chosen as being likely to first be hypnotized and second to respond to suggestions. These 57 individuals were then screened for brain activity using magnetic resonance imaging (MRI), which is used to measure the flow of blood throughout the body and to the brain. After their initial screening, the patients were ready to be hypnotized (Jiang et al., 2017).

The subjects were first told to move their eyes around, turn their gaze upward, then close their eyes. They were then instructed to let their muscles soften as if they were floating in a great lake; then, they were told to think of how it feels to be happy by either thinking of a memory of a vacation or something similar. After following a series of hypnosis exercises, the subjects then had to undergo an eight-minute brain scan. The results found that the patients' connectivity between the dorsolateral prefrontal cortex and insula was significantly stronger. These are the regions of the brain governing body control, emotions, empathy, memory, and decision making. Participants also found that there was a decreased connection in the brain's default mode, which is where we are found to constantly think about ourselves and our actions. Overall, the study revealed that under hypnosis, the brain is able to detach from the ego and view situations, memories, events, and people from an outside and from a more logical perspective (Jiang et al., 2017).

While it can be seemingly impossible to describe sensations under hypnosis, there are a few things that almost all people who receive hypnosis experience. The first is, as we mentioned previously, relaxation. This not only involves muscle and physical relaxation but also a sense of ease for the mind. It can slow or stop a mind that is racing, chatting, or in constant attentiveness so it can experience calm. The patient might feel extremely heavy, the eyes might feel very droopy, and they may find themselves simply unable to think complex thoughts. It is very important to note that this is actually not the hypnosis that is causing this sensation but rather your brain responding to the hypnotherapist's suggestions. The patient is the one relaxing their body and mind yourself, proving that humans actually have absolute control over our mind and body if we can reach that state. Many patients also experience a sense of ultimate focus and concentration. Individuals have found their mind is focused on the present moment and will not wander as it so often usually does. Since the hypnotherapist is guiding the patient, they will probably be attentive to everything they say and not want to even think of anything else. There is also an acute sense of open-mindedness. You may feel more open to suggestions and advice and to seeing things in different ways. You may also find yourself detached from emotions and objective feelings.

When it comes to anxiety, while the conscious mind might remember every little detail of trauma or map out every little detail of something going wrong, it cannot detect exactly how it affects us. When there are too many things to process, details are often stored away from the conscious mind, and some are repressed, an innate form of self-care, so we consciously don't have to deal with everything. However, that doesn't mean they still aren't deeply impacting us in nearly everything we do and how we live.

During a hypnotic session, you'll be given the chance to go back and visualize the times you have previously experienced anxiety. Maybe you'll find that your feelings of anxiety stem from a particular activity, such as falling or being rejected. In the same breath, by using hypnoprojectives, you can undergo a process of visualizing past events as you would have liked them to have occurred. Then you can witness your future and take action in a more calming manner, facing your fears head-on and headstrong.

Hypnosis can be an extremely effective, if not the most effective, tool to realize and release these hidden details that are subconsciously causing us pain and anxiety. It gives the mind the ability to transport through the space of time and go to unexplored parts of the brain so we can fully examine what is negatively affecting our being. It opens the door that leads to a room of unwanted memories—the memories that are making us suffer in the present. Only once we fully tap into the source, analyze the root cause, and deal with these traumatic memories we begin the process of true healing.

The hypnotherapy healing process eliminates the undesired pain caused from these repressed memories and emotions. It unblocks that which has created a barrier between your current experience and living a healthy, happy, and full life. This healing process may require numerous therapy sessions, but it's a very important first step in truly living in your present life and not being ambushed by deep seeded issues from your past.

Examples Of A Hypnotherapy Session

We do not recommend hypnotherapy for anyone who has had a psychotic episode or for anyone using drugs or alcohol on a regular basis.

A hypnotherapy session begins with the therapist asking the patient a series of questions and conducting a brief analysis. This is what is referred to as talk therapy. It can help a patient process their thoughts and situations, all while offering them comfort and trust. Then, the patient will be transported into a trance, which, as we have learned, is a state of acute subconscious awareness. This trance feels different to everyone and therefore does not have an umbrella concept that can describe the exact feeling or sensations of being hypnotized. However, it can be said that the patient will feel completely relaxed and free from any stresses or feelings of anxiety. The hypnotherapist will return you to your original state and complete the session with another conversation.

There are a few things to keep in mind if you want to give hypnotherapy a go: Find a hypnotist you trust by conducting research, going for appointments, and speaking to others who have been to a hypnotherapist. When you meet a hypnotherapist, ask them about their training and certification. Once you've found someone you trust, come up with a treatment plan, then begin your healing process knowing you are in control of your session. You still have freewill intact, and you will not be made to do anything against your will that can shame you in any way. A hypnotherapy session is intended to be a safe space. This is not the kind of activity you see on TV or at a magic show. If you ever have doubts, remember why you started, and know that helping yourself is the first step for the process to work and the true healing to begin.

Hypnotherapy has been proven to be an incredibly useful and effective tool to heal trauma, pain, and anxiety, as well as ward off addictions and bad habits, creating new ones in their place. Always make sure you are with a professional when undergoing hypnosis. Whatever level of anxiety you live with it can be useful to integrate Hypnotherapy to identify and address the source of your issues. Hypnotherapy is known to generate numerous benefits. It helps focus the mind, ease both physical and emotional tension, relaxes the body, and aids in gaining a deeper sense of emotional control. If you suffer from severe anxiety or post-traumatic stress disorder, hypnotherapy could be the tool that helps you find freedom and live your best life.

Reflection

Have you experienced a psychotic episode, or do you use drugs or alcohol on a regular basis? If yes, please do not try hypnotherapy, use a different modality to assist you in managing your anxiety. If no, is hypnotherapy a modality you would like to consider?

- Have you tried other healing techniques that have not worked, to overcome your anxiety?

- Do you consider your anxiety to be deep, extreme, or chronic?

- Are you willing to trust a licensed hypnotherapist?

- List resources where you can identify hypnotherapists to evaluate.

- What will you measure to identify the value and impact of the sessions?

Notes & things to remember....

CHAPTER TEN

CONCLUSION

You deserve to have options to manage all the different ways anxiety shows up in your life. We have provided you some incredible alternative healing methods to try, in conjunction with or in lieu of medication. Millions of people are struggling with their anxiety and having skills to manage such a hardship is inspiring. Every move or thought inflicted with anxiety can have huge impacts on your daily life. Alternative medicine is not always the first thought that may come to your mind. Hopefully this book helped you learn a bit more about yourself and identified useful tools to consider, that may be more powerful than you realized.

Laughter releases chemicals in our brain that have antianxiety effects, decreases the production of the stress hormone cortisol, and invites your body to relax, allowing us to reduce stress, anxiety and increase serotonin levels. Exercise also releases endorphins and chemicals in the brain that trigger a calming response, causing us to relax. If done over an extended period of time, exercise can help us prepare our bodies to better handle future periods of stress. Ayurveda takes a mind, body, and spirit approach through ancient techniques that may create a balanced life with minimal stress and anxiety. While incorporating aromatherapy uses the healing properties of thousands of plant-based oils to soothe or awaken the nervous system, amygdala region of the brain, and the immune functions of the body.

Animal therapy allows you to create a bond with an animal, which provides a sense of closeness, belonging, and allows for a physical and emotional shift where you can lower your walls and release the tension and anxiety you carry. Energy therapy, opens blockages within your chakras, allowing you to release tension, let your energy flow freely, finding balance so your body can heal itself. Sound therapy uses frequencies to elevate your mind away from your everyday thoughts to bring you to a peaceful place, allowing you to release your anxiety and be at peace in the moment. Finally, hypnotherapy allows you to find the root cause of your anxiety and provides a hypnotic approach to address and overcome it.

Some of these modalities are very simple and easy to apply to your everyday life. Laughter, sound, and exercise are great therapies that you can do on your own. Other modalities such as essential oils, yoga or Ayurveda would prove more beneficial with guidance from a practitioner.

Alternative medicine offers proven modalities to consider integrating into your life so that you can find relief and freedom. We encourage you to take the time to select two of these alternative therapies. Integrate them into your daily life and schedule. Make sure to track which approach is providing you the most benefits. Check the addendum to create something useful or buy and customize the *What Makes Me Feel Better?* workbook. Over time, look at including another form of therapy from the list. We are all different, so it may take some trial and error to find the right mix of therapies for you.

Living with anxiety, lack of sleep, concentration loss, muscle tension, and racing mind creates an uncomfortable and limited life. There is an old saying, "Stop doing what doesn't work." The other side of this idea is, "Keep doing what works." Identify where you are today and be clear of what getting healthier looks like for you personally. Let your body heal itself as you integrate holistic healing to take charge of your circumstances and create a happy, healthy life.

— • —

WHAT MAKES ME FEEL BETTER?

We hope you live a happy, healthy life by continuing to do what works. Being open to trying new medicine whether alternative or prescribed can be a commitment to bettering your life. The opportunity to track what works and what doesn't work is a gift we are giving you. The question then becomes, how are you measuring what works and what doesn't? When people ask you how you are and your response is, "fine," or "okay," there is no certainty and no clarity of how you actually are.

Once you begin integrating a prescription from your doctor or one of the alternative healing options in this book, we encourage you to get to know yourself better and decide what is helpful and what is not.

Create your tracking form by using a spreadsheet, an online file, jot it down on a piece of paper, or order What Makes Me Feel Better? workbook from Choosing Goodness on Amazon.

1. Across the top, choose four areas of your life that are currently impacted by your anxiety. Body, Mind, Heart, and Spirit are a place to start.

2. Specify the scale for each of those areas as a note in a spreadsheet, on a second page of a computer document, or on the back of a piece of paper.

3. Write the date in the left column.

4. Every day, at the same time(s), evaluate the impact the medicine is having, so you know for yourself if your life is changing and how.

Create a scale to evaluate the impact of the medicine you are integrating into your life. Medical environments often ask patients to use a scale of 1-10 to describe their pain, energy level, or other issues. When creating a scale we encourage an even number of options so you cannot choose the middle number. Daily you get to decide if your current situation is in the healthier range or still needs improvement. Review the questions below and use the possible scales as examples. Add what comes to mind if there is nothing on the list that you feel is relevant for your health and wellness.

The goal is to learn about yourself and be able to identify ways you are getting healthier so you can continue your healing journey with tools / medicine you know are effective for you, because you measured it.

EXAMPLES OF PERSONAL WELLBEING SCALES

Here are examples of themes and scales for you to consider, or modify, to personalize your evaluation.

Body - How is anxiety showing up in my body?

Joint flexibility

4 = Unlimited flexibility

3 = Moving and it aches

2 = Stiff, a little flexibility

1 = Stationary, immobile, no flexibility

Ability to Move Freely

4 = Total physical freedom

3 = Some movement even if I'm sore

2 = Moving, even though it is painful

1 = Chronic pain, it hurts to move

Physical strength

4 = Strong

3 = Building strength

2 = Testing my strength

1 = Weak

Mind - How is anxiety impacting my mind?

Mental judgment

4 = Peaceful, no judgment

3 = Able to release judgment quickly

2 = Intermittent judgment

1 = Constant judgement

How calm is my mind?

4 = Calm mind

3 = Mind is inconsistently calm

2 = Brain fog, my mind is a little busy

1 = Racing mind, debilitating

Impact of my thoughts

4 = Consistently grateful, kind and appreciative thoughts

3 = Intermittent positive and appreciative thoughts

2 = Thinking about what to appreciate, easier to appreciate others than myself

1 = Mean and unkind thoughts

Heart / Emotions - How does anxiety feel in my heart?

Am I joyful?

4 = Joyful

3 = Mindful with bits of joy

2 = Sad

1 = Depressed

How is my ability to feel love?

4 = Feeling loved and sharing love

3 = Noticing some compassion

2 = Some connection, sometimes disconnected

1 = Isolated

Do I feel fulfilled?

4 = Feeling fulfilled and worthy

3 = Doing the work, seeing the light

2 = Struggling with what I want to do

1 = Traumatized

Spirit/ Connection to high power - How is anxiety impacting my spirit / energy?

Am I playful?

4 = I am playful

3 = My energy feels lighter and I laugh

2 = My energy feels burdened, I have some breaks

1 = My energy feels heavy and weighs me down

Am I hopeful?

4 = I am hopeful

3 = I am practicing believing in myself and others

2 = My energy feels resistant

1 = My energy feels stressed

Am I connected to a higher source of energy?

4 = I am comfortable and connecting to a higher source

3 = I am practicing trust of myself and others

2 = my energy feels nervous

1 = my energy feels terrified

Consider other areas to measure: personal energy, talking with others, creative time, helping another, eating healthy....

— • —

2 WEEK IMPACT OF COMPLEMENTARY HEALING

Here is an example of how this tracking approach measurements actions and impact for 2 weeks. You can create this in an electronic spreadsheet, in a table in Word, on a piece of paper, or look for the *What Makes Me Feel Better?* workbook from Choosing Goodness.

Medicine	Body	Mind	Heart	Spirit
60 second Laughing meditation every morning. Animal Therapy every Mon & Wed 60 minutes QiGong 2 times a week	**Joint Flexibility** 4=unlimited flexibility 3=moving and it aches 2=stiff, a little flexibility 1=stationary, immobile, no flexibility	**Calm mind** 4=Calm mind 3=mind is inconsistently calm 2=some brain fog, some busy mind 1=racing mind, debilitating	**Ability to feel Love** 4=Feeling loved and sharing love 3=compassionate, engaging 2=a bit of connection, sometimes disconnected 1=isolated	**Playful** 4=I am playful 3=my energy feels lighter and I laugh 2=my energy feels burdened, I have some breaks 1=my energy feels heavy and weighed down
8/1/2020	1	1	1	1
8/2/2020	1	1	1	1
8/3/2020	2	1	1	2
8/4/2020	2	2	1	2
8/5/2020	2	2	2	2
8/6/2020	2	2	2	2
8/7/2020	2	2	2	3
8/8/2020	3	2	2	3
8/9/2020	3	2	2	3
8/10/2020	3	3	2	3
8/11/2020	3	3	2	3
8/12/2020	2	3	2	4
8/13/2020	2	2	2	4
8/14/2020	2	3	3	4
8/15/2020	3	4	3	4

References

8 Benefits of Reiki Healing. (2020, January 10). Mindset First. https://mindsetfirst.ca/8-benefits-of-reiki-healing/

About Us. (2021, September 20). Retrieved from Havin' a Laugh Charity: https://www.havinalaugh.com/about/

Akimbekov, N. S., & Razzaque, M. S. (2021). Laughter therapy: A humor-induced hormonal intervention to reduce stress and anxiety. Retrieved from ScienceDirect: https://www.sciencedirect.com/science/article/pii/S266594412100016X

Ali, B., Al-Wabel, N. A., Shams, S., Ahamad, A., Khan, S. A., & Anwar, F. (2015). Essential oils used in aromatherapy: A systemic review. Asian Pacific Journal of Tropical Biomedicine, 5(8), 601–611. https://doi.org/10.1016/j.apjtb.2015.05.007

Anderson, C. (2016, August 2). I Didn't Leave My House For An Entire Year—Until Fitness Saved My Life. Shape. https://www.shape.com/lifestyle/mind-and-body/how-i-overcame-anxiety-disorder

Anxiety and Depression Association of America. (2000). Exercise for Stress and Anxiety | Anxiety and Depression Association of America, ADAA. Adaa.org. https://adaa.org/living-with-anxiety/managing-anxiety/exercise-stress-and-anxiety

Authentic Ayurvedic Treatments In Kerala, India. (n.d.). Retrieved 2021, from Somatheeram Ayurvedic Health Resort: https://somatheeram.org/en/

Ayurveda. (2019). Johns Hopkins Medicine. https://www.hopkinsmedicine.org/health/wellness-and-prevention/ayurveda

Barati, F., Nasiri, A., Akbari, N., & Sharifzadeh, G. (2016). The Effect of Aromatherapy on Anxiety in (Facts & Statistics, n.d.) Patients. Nephro-Urology Monthly, 8(5). https://doi.org/10.5812/numonthly.38347

Bauman, D. (2020, April 16). Sound Therapy: A Source of Comfort and Healing During Pandemic. Spectrumlocalnews.com. https://spectrumlocalnews.com/tx/san-antonio/news/2020/04/16/sound-therapy--a-source-of-comfort-and-healing-during-pandemic

Bertone, H. (2020, October 2). 6 Types of Meditation: Which One Is Right for You? Healthline. https://www.healthline.com/health/mental-health/types-of-meditation#benefits

Budd, K. (2019, September 11). An Ayurvedic Approach to Anxiety. Chopra. https://chopra.com/articles/an-ayurvedic-approach-to-anxiety

College, A. &. (2017, September 19). Meridians in Traditional Chinese Medicine? | AMC-Miami, Florida. Retrieved from Acupuncture

Massage College:
https://www.amcollege.edu/blog/what-are-meridians-in-traditional-ch
inese-medicine-tcm

Costello, Yolanda Saez. (2020, May 14). Tapping for Child Anxiety: A
Personal Story. The Tapping Solution.
https://www.thetappingsolution.com/blog/tapping-for-child-anxiety-
a-personal-story/

Cromwell, M. (2015, April 1). The
History of Sound Healing. MASSAGE Magazine.
https://www.massagemag.com/the-history-of-sound-healing-29245/

Cronkleton, E. (2019, March 8). What Is Aromatherapy and How Does
It Help Me? Healthline.
https://www.healthline.com/health/what-is-aromatherapy#how-does-i
t-work?

Cuncic, A. (2019a). Top Reasons to Take Part in Animal-Assisted
Therapy for SAD. Verywell Mind.
https://www.verywellmind.com/animal-assisted-therapy-for-social-anx
iety-disorder-4049422

Cuncic, A. (2019b). Top Tips to Use Essential Oils for Social Anxiety.
Verywell Mind.
https://www.verywellmind.com/how-is-aromatherapy-used-for-social-
anxiety-disorder-3024210

Davidson, K. (2021, January 8). Laughing Yoga: What
Is It and Does It Work? Retrieved from Healthline:
https://www.healthline.com/nutrition/laughing-yoga#how-to-do-it

Del Turco, L. (2019, October 7). I Was Skeptical About Reiki — And Then I Tried It for My Anxiety. Greatist. https://greatist.com/live/i-tried-reiki#Skeptic

Demant, J. (n.d.). History of Hypnotherapy and Hypnosis. Retrieved September 24, 2021, from Jason Demant. https://jasondemant.com/history-of-hypnotherapy-and-hypnosis/]

Directors., Developed through collaboration and consensus by the Healing Beyond Borders (HBB) Education Committee and approved by the HBB Board of. (2010). HTI Healing Touch Certification Programs Level 1 Student Workbook. Lakewood, CO, USA: Healing Touch International, Inc (HTI).

Erika. (2020, July 30). 7 Best Exercises for Anxiety and Depression. Talking Circles Therapy & Wellness, LLC. https://talkingcirclestherapy.com/7-best-exercises-for-anxiety-and-depression/

Estrada, J. (2020, March 26). 3 ways to bring your body vibrational balance using sound healing therapy. Well+Good. https://www.wellandgood.com/sound-healing/

Everything About Emotional Support Animals. (n.d.). Retrieved 2021, from American Kennel Club: https://www.akc.org/expert-advice/news/everything-about-emotional-support-animals/

Facts & Statistics. (n.d.). Retrieved from Anxiety & Depression Association of America: https://adaa.org/understanding-anxiety/facts-statistics

Fisher, C. (2015, April 30). Reiki and psychotherapy. Counseling Today. https://ct.counseling.org/2015/04/reiki-and-psychotherapy/#

Flanagan, D. (n.d.). Reiki: Gentle Yet Powerful Anxiety Relief. Anxiety.org. Retrieved July 21, 2021, from https://www.anxiety.org/reiki-anxiety-relief-gentle-powerful-way-allevi ate-anxiety

Force, N. (2018, December 9). Laugh in the Face of Anxiety. Psych Central. https://psychcentral.com/lib/laugh-in-the-face-of-anxiety#1

Friedman, R. S., Burg, M. M., Miles, P., Lee, F., & Lampert, R. (2010). Effects of Reiki on autonomic activity early after acute coronary syndrome. Journal of the American College of Cardiology, 56(12), 995-996.

Frisch, N. (2001, May 31). Nursing as a Context for Alternative/Complementary Modalities. 6(2). Retrieved from OJIN The Online Journal of Issues In Nursing: https://ojin.nursingworld.org/MainMenuCategories/ANAMarketplac e/ANAPeriodicals/OJIN/TableofContents/Volume62001/No2May0 1/AlternativeComplementaryModalities.html

Goodreads. (n.d.). Quote by Jack Kornfield. Goodreads. https://www.goodreads.com/quotes/7243963-may-i-be-filled-with-lov ing-kindness-may-i-be-well

Halpern, M. (2007, August 28). Ayurveda and Asana: Yoga Poses for Your Health. Retrieved from Yoga Journal: https://www.yogajournal.com/lifestyle/health/ayurveda-and-asana/

Hartney, E. (2020, November 17). What Does Hypnosis Feel Like? Verywell Mind. https://www.verywellmind.com/what-does-hypnosis-feel-like-4141150

Healing Beyond Borders Education Committee. (2010) Healing Touch Certificate Program Level 1 Student Workbook. .

Healing Beyond Borders. (n.d.). Retrieved from Healing Beyond Borders: www.healingbeyondborders.org

Historical Background and Evolution of Physical Activity Recommendations | Surgeon General Report. (2020). Centers for Disease Control and Prevention. https://www.cdc.gov/nccdphp/sgr/intro2.htm

How TAPPING Can Help Reduce Stress & Anxiety About Coronavirus. (2020, March 25). Retrieved from YouTube: https://www.youtube.com/watch?v=d3XiDmhrxLk

How to Tap with Jessica Ortner: Emotional Freedom Technique Informational Video. (2013, April 11). Retrieved from YouTube: https://www.youtube.com/watch?v=pAclBdj20ZU

Hopkins, J. (n.d.). History of Sound Healing. Retrieved September 24 2021, from Red Doors Studio: https://www.red-doors.com/sound-healing

Hoshaw, C. (2020, June 1). What Can Ayurveda Teach Us About Anxiety? Healthline. https://www.healthline.com/health/10-steps-to-still-anxiety-according -to-ayurveda#Fortify-your-system

Howley, E. K. (2020). 12 Best Exercises to Ease Stress and Anxiety. US News & World Report; U.S. News & World Report. https://health.usnews.com/health-care/patient-advice/articles/best-exe rcises-to-ease-stress-and-anxiety

Hypnosis. (2021, July 21). In Wikipedia. https://en.wikipedia.org/wiki/Hypnosis

Jaiswal, Y. S., & Williams, L. L. (2017). A glimpse of Ayurveda –
The forgotten history and principles of Indian traditional medicine.
Journal of Traditional and Complementary Medicine, 7(1), 50–53.
https://doi.org/10.1016/j.jtcme.2016.02.002

Jiang, H., White, M. P., Greicius, M. D., Waelde, L. C., & Spiegel, D.
(2017). Brain Activity and Functional Connectivity Associated with
Hypnosis. Cerebral cortex (New York, N.Y. : 1991), 27(8), 4083–4093.
https://doi.org/10.1093/cercor/bhw220

John, R. (2014, June). Hypnotic Regression and Healing the
Unconscious Mind. Psychology Today.
https://www.psychologytoday.com/us/blog/hypnosis-the-power-tranc
e/201406/hypnotic-regression-and-healing-the-unconscious-mind

Johnson, J. (2020, July 10). Animal therapy: How
it works, benefits, and more. Www.medicalnewstoday.com.
https://www.medicalnewstoday.com/articles/animal-therapy#benefits

Jiu, Z. Z., Zhou, X.-F., Li, Y., Zhu, H., & Chen, L.-L. (2013, May).
Impacts of acupuncture at twelve meridians acupoints on brain waves
of patients with general anxiety disorder. Retrieved from PubMed.com:
https://pubmed.ncbi.nlm.nih.gov/23885609/

Kaplan, I. (2017, August 28). I Didn't Believe Hypnosis
Could Work — Until It Changed My Life. Allure.
https://www.allure.com/story/hypnosis-anxiety-depression-treatment

Klein, G. J., Krouse, M., & Lowe, K. (2014, July 26). Using
Healing Touch to Help Junior Nursing Students with Their Anxiety.
Retrieved from 25th International Nursing Research Congress:
https://stti.confex.com/stti/congrs14/webprogram/Paper66977.html

Laughter Yoga Health Craze Sweeping the World. (2021, September 20). Retrieved from Laughter Yoga University: https://laughteryoga.org/

Louie, D., Brook, K., & Frates, E. (2016). The Laughter Prescription. American Journal of Lifestyle Medicine, 10(4), 262–267. https://doi.org/10.1177/1559827614550279

Mackintosh, G., & Stapleton, P. B. (2020). Ep 3: Dr. Peta Stapleton-The Science Behind Tapping. Bond University. https://research.bond.edu.au/en/publications/ep-3-dr-peta-stapleton-the-science-behind-tapping

Majumdar, M. (2018, June 14). Seven Chakras and Our Health-(Muladhara to Sahasrara. Retrieved from MedIndia: https://www.medindia.net/patients/lifestyleandwellness/seven-chakras-and-our-health.htm

Mandal, A. (2018, August 23). Acupuncture History. News-Medical.net. https://www.news-medical.net/health/Acupuncture-History.aspx

McKusick, E. D. (2020). The Human Biofield. Retrieved from Chiropractic Newsletter Well-Being: https://drmcatamney.com/uploads/Well-Being_The+Human+Biofield[1].pdf

McPherson, K. (2021, April 21). EFT tapping for relief from stress and anxiety. ANMJ. https://anmj.org.au/eft-tapping-for-relief-from-stress-and-anxiety/

Monroe, R. (2017, October 2). How Essential Oils Became the Cure for Our Age of Anxiety. The New Yorker. https://www.newyorker.com/magazine/2017/10/09/how-essential-oils-became-the-cure-for-our-age-of-anxiety

Morrison, M. L. (2007). Health Benefits of Animal-Assisted Interventions. Complementary Health Practice Review, 12(1), 51–62. https://doi.org/10.1177/1533210107302397

Nanda, A. (n.d.). The 7 Chakra: Know the Seven Chakra Life energy. Retrieved September 22, 2021, from Moksha Mantra: https://www.mokshamantra.com/7-chakras-know-seven-chakras/

NEUROLOGIC MUSIC THERAPY. (n.d.). Retrieved September 22, 2021, from NMTSA Neurologic Music Therapy Services of Arizona: https://www.nmtsa.org/what-is-nmt

Newman, T. (2018, September 5). Is anxiety increasing in the United States? Www.medicalnewstoday.com. https://www.medicalnewstoday.com/articles/322877

Nick Ortner's Tapping Technique to Calm Anxiety & Stress in 3 Minutes. (2020, October 29). Retrieved from YouTube: https://www.youtube.com/watch?v=02bN4JFx10Y

Nordoff-Robbins Center for Music Therapy. (n.d.). Retrieved September 22, 2021, from NYU/Steinhardt: https://steinhardt.nyu.edu/nordoff/the-practice

Ortner, A. (2020). Tapping for Child Anxiety: A Personal Story. The Tapping Solution.https://www.thetappingsolution.com/blog/tapping-for-child-anxiety-a-personal-story/

Pet Partners. (2021). Retrieved from Pet Partners: https://petpartners.org/

Petitt, T. (2020, April 16). Sound Therapy: A Source of Comfort and Healing During Pandemic. Spectrum News 1.

https://spectrumlocalnews.com/tx/san-antonio/news/2020/04/16/so
und-therapy--a-source-of-comfort-and-healing-during-pandemic

Physical Fitness: Its History, Evolution, and Future | The Art of
Manliness. (2018, October 23). The Art of Manliness.
https://www.artofmanliness.com/articles/the-history-of-physical-fitnes
s/

Purtill, (2016, January 20). Turns out "sound healing" can be actually,
well, healing. Quartz.
https://qz.com/595315/turns-out-sound-healing-can-be-actually-well-
healing/

QuoteFancy. (n.d.). Pythagoras Quote. QuoteFancy.
https://quotefancy.com/quote/1374655/Pythagoras-Each-celestial-bo
dy-in-fact-each-and-every-atom-produces-a-particular-sound-on

Rand, W. L. (2000). Reiki - The Healing Touch. Vision Publications.

Rand, W.L. (n.d). The Greatest Healing the World has Known.
https://www.reiki.org/articles/greatest-healing-world-has-known

Ratey, J. J. (2019, October 24). Can exercise help treat anxiety? - Harvard
Health Blog. Harvard Health Blog.
https://www.health.harvard.edu/blog/can-exercise-help-treat-anxiety-2
019102418096

Robinson, L. (2018). How to Start Exercising and Stick to It: Making
Exercise an Enjoyable Part of Your Everyday Life. Helpguide.org.
https://www.helpguide.org/articles/healthy-living/how-to-start-exercis
ing-and-stick-to-it.htm

Robinson, L. (2020, October). Laughter is the Best Medicine -
HelpGuide.org. Https://Www.helpguide.org.

https://www.helpguide.org/articles/mental-health/laughter-is-the-best -medicine.htm#

Rodriguez, D. (2009, June 2).
Anti-Anxiety Workout. EverydayHealth.com.
https://www.everydayhealth.com/anxiety/anxiety-and-exercise.aspx

Santos-Longhurst, A. (2020, January 27). The
Uses and Benefits of Music Therapy. Healthline.
https://www.healthline.com/health/sound-healing

Schwartz, A. (n.d.). The Story of A Psychiatric Service Dog Team - Information on Anxiety and Other Anxiety Related Mental Health Disorders. Mental Help.
https://www.mentalhelp.net/blogs/the-story-of-a-psychiatric-service-d og-team/

Semeco, A. (2017, February 10). The Top 10 Benefits of Regular Exercise. Healthline.
https://www.healthline.com/nutrition/10-benefits-of-exercise#TOC_ TITLE_HDR_10

Service, emotional support, and therapy animals. (n.d.). Retrieved 2021, from AVMA American Veterinary Medical Association:
https://www.avma.org/resources-tools/animal-health-welfare/service-e motional-support-and-therapy-animals

Shah, P. (2020, August 20). A Primer of the Chakra System. Retrieved from Chopra: https://chopra.com/articles/what-is-a-chakra

Shamini, J., McMahon, G. F., Hansen, P., Kozub, M. P., Porter, V., King, R., & Guarneri, E. M. (2012, September). Healing Touch With Guided Imagery for PTSD in Returning Active Duty Military: A Randomized

Controlled Trial. Military Medicine, 177(9), 1015-1021. Retrieved from https://doi.org/10.7205/MILMED-D-11-00290

Smith, B. (2016, July 31). This is your brain under hypnosis. Cosmos Magazine. https://cosmosmagazine.com/biology/this-is-what-happens-to-your-brain-under-hypnosis/

Sound Therapy. (n.d.). Retrieved September 24, 2021, from Holistic Healing Therapy: http://holistichealingtherapy.co.uk/sound-therapy/sound-therapy-history/

Spoor, P. S., & Swift, G. W. (2000). The Huygens entrainment phenomenon and thermoacoustic engines. The Journal of the Acoustical Society of America, 108(2), 588–599. https://doi.org/10.1121/1.429590

Staff, H. (2020, September 23). Therapeutic Touch. Retrieved from University of Michigan Health: https://www.uofmhealth.org/health-library/ag2078spec

Stanborough, R. (2020, November 13). What Is Vibrational Energy? Definition, Benefits & More. Healthline. https://www.healthline.com/health/vibrational-energy#what-we-know

Stelter, G. (2016, October 4). Chakras: A Beginner's Guide to the 7 Chakras. Healthline. https://www.healthline.com/health/fitness-exercise/7-chakras#The-takeaway

Tang, S. K., & Tse, M. Y. (2014). Aromatherapy: does it help to relieve pain, depression, anxiety, and stress in community-dwelling older persons?. BioMed research international, 2014, 430195. https://doi.org/10.1155/2014/430195

Tapping 101 - Learn the Basics of the Tapping Technique. (n.d.). Www.thetappingsolution.com. https://www.thetappingsolution.com/tapping-101/

The 12 Major Meridians. (2020, October 12). Retrieved from Danai Wellness: https://danaiwellness.com/the-12-major-meridians/

The Origin and Causes of the Opioid Epidemic. (2018, August 14). Retrieved from Georgetown Behavioral Health Institute: https://www.georgetownbehavioral.com/blog/origin-and-causes-of-op ioid-epidemic

Thoma, M. V., La Marca, R., Brönnimann, R., Finkel, L., Ehlert, U., & Nater, U. M. (2013). The Effect of Music on the Human Stress Response. PLoS ONE, 8(8), e70156. https://doi.org/10.1371/journal.pone.0070156

Twelve Main Meridians in traditional Chinese medicine. (2014, January 30) VedaPulse.com. https://vedapulse.com/twelve-main-meridians-in-traditional-chinese-medicine

Ulrich R. S. (1984). View through a window may influence recovery from surgery. Science (New York, N.Y.), 224(4647), 420–421. https://doi.org/10.1126/science.6143402

Vidrascu, E. (2018, August 15). Sound Healing for Treatment of Chronic Pain, Anxiety, Stress, and Drug Addiction, Part 1: An Introduction. JPHMP Direct. https://jphmpdirect.com/2018/08/15/sound-healing-and-therapy-for-

treatment-of-pain-anxiety-stress-and-drug-addiction-part-1-an-introdu
ction/

Waynne, A. (2017, September 15). Can
Energy Healing Cure Anxiety? Www.healyourlife.com.
https://www.healyourlife.com/can-energy-healing-cure-anxiety

What Are Psychiatric Service Dogs? (2020). Retrieved from WebMD:
https://www.webmd.com/anxiety-panic/what-are-psychiatric-service-d
ogs

What is the U.S. Opioid Epidemic? (2021, February 19).
Retrieved from U.S. Departement of Health and Human Services:
https://www.hhs.gov/opioids/about-the-epidemic/index.html

West, H. (2019, September 30). What Are Essential Oils, and Do They
Work? Healthline; Healthline Media.
https://www.healthline.com/nutrition/what-are-essential-oils#what-th
ey-are

Wide Open Pets. (2021). Retrieved from Wide Open Pets:
https://www.wideopenpets.com/

Wong, C. (2021, February 26). How Emotions and Organs Are
Connected in Traditional Chinese Medicine.
https://www.verywellmind.com/emotions-in-traditional-chinese-medi
cine-88196

Woodford, C. (2019, February 20). Sound - The science of
waves, how they travel, how we use them. Explain That Stuff.
https://www.explainthatstuff.com/sound.html

Yazdani, M., Esmaeilzadeh, M., Pahlavanzadeh, S., & Khaledi, F. (2014). The effect of laughter Yoga on general health among nursing students. Iranian journal of nursing and midwifery research, 19(1), 36–40.

Yim, J. (2016). Therapeutic Benefits of Laughter in Mental Health: A Theoretical Review. The Tohoku Journal of Experimental Medicine, 239(3), 243–249. https://doi.org/10.1620/tjem.239.243

Yoga and Ayurveda. (n.d.). Retrieved September 22, 2021, from Banyan Botanicals: https://www.banyanbotanicals.com/info/ayurvedic-living/living-ayurveda/yoga/

ABOUT THE AUTHOR

After receiving a bachelors degree in Agricultural and Managerial Economics in 1981, P. Restaino worked at various sized corporations for over twenty five years. Her lessons included learning to cooperate with people from experiences in sales, marketing, project management, training, and leadership.

Working with non-profits fueled her passion as she facilitated courses that empowered women; assisted creating a world where youth are safe, loved and celebrated; produced annual queer dance competitions; organized volunteers at events that generated donations or a magical experience for all.

P. Restaino earned a Masters of Arts in Socio-Cultural Anthropology in 2009. Teaching life skills to first year students at California State University, East Bay for 6 years, her facilitation techniques shifted to be more interactive and engaging while she learned to appreciate another generation.

Two of her favorite things in life are letting her excitement overflow when she watches women's basketball. The second is traveling to other countries and experience how beautiful it is to feel people around the world share their richness through music, dance, creative expression, food, and gatherings.

Sharing Healing Touch, a heart-centered, energy modality is a gift. Her work is to balance her client's body, mind, heart, and spirit, in a healing way. She is learning about the Ayurveda philosophy, as well as ancient medicine from indigenous grandmothers, and Aztec friends. P. Restaino is known to collaborate with alternative medicine practitioners whenever possible.

Additional Books to Consider Reading

I decided to share some books I found interesting and insightful to read:

Healing from Family Trauma

A Guidebook for Adult Children of Toxic Parents

by Christine A. Fisher, BSN, RNC

ISBN 9798834809678   ASIN B0B385V7F9

This book is packed with advice, guidance, and proactive actions you can take to cope with childhood traumas and leave them where they belong ...In the past!

Braiding Sweetgrass

Indigenous Wisdom, Scientific Knowledge, and the Teachings of Plants

by Robin Wall Kimmerer

ISBN 9781571313560   ASIN B01H4772CU

Only when we can hear the languages of other beings are we capable of understanding the generosity of the earth, and learning to give our own gifts in return.

The Book of Joy

Lasting Happiness in a Changing World

by His Holiness the Dalai Lama, Archbishop Desmond Tutu, Douglas Abrams

Read or listen to what is shared as the Dalai Lama and Desmond Tutu explore the nature of true joy and confront each of the obstacles to joy – from fear, stress, and anger to grief, illness and death. They then offer us the eight pillars of Joy, which provide the foundation for lasting happiness.

ISBN 9780399185045   Online availability
https://www.penguinrandomhouse.com/books/533718

Made in United States
North Haven, CT
15 October 2023

42761190R00091